EVERY WOMAN'S GUIDE TO HEART HEALTH

JILL ECKERSLEY is a freelance writer with many years' experience of writing on health topics. She is a regular contributor to women's and general-interest magazines, including *Good Health*, *Bella*, *Ms London*, *Goodtimes*, *Slimming World* and other titles. *Coping with Snoring and Sleep Apnoea*, *Coping with Childhood Asthma*, *Coping with Dyspraxia*, *Coping with Childhood Allergies* and *Helping Children Cope with Anxiety*, five books written by Jill for Sheldon Press, were all published in 2003–6. She lives beside the Regent's Canal in north London with two cats.

Overcoming Common Problems Series

Selected titles
A full list of titles is available from Sheldon Press,
36 Causton Street, London SW1P 4ST, and on our website at
www.sheldonpress.co.uk

Assertiveness: Step by Step
Dr Windy Dryden and Daniel Constantinou

Breaking Free
Carolyn Ainscough and Kay Toon

Calm Down
Paul Hauck

Cataract: What You Need to Know
Mark Watts

Cider Vinegar
Margaret Hills

Comfort for Depression
Janet Horwood

Confidence Works
Gladeana McMahon

Coping Successfully with Pain
Neville Shone

Coping Successfully with Panic-Attacks
Shirley Trickett

Coping Successfully with Period Problems
Mary-Claire Mason

Coping Successfully with Prostate Cancer
Dr Tom Smith

Coping Successfully with Ulcerative Colitis
Peter Cartwright

Coping Successfully with Your Hiatus Hernia
Dr Tom Smith

Coping Successfully with Your Irritable Bowel
Rosemary Nicol

Coping with Alopecia
Dr Nigel Hunt and Dr Sue McHale

Coping with Anxiety and Depression
Shirley Trickett

Coping with Blushing
Dr Robert Edelmann

Coping with Bowel Cancer
Dr Tom Smith

Coping with Brain Injury
Maggie Rich

Coping with Candida
Shirley Trickett

Coping with Chemotherapy
Dr Terry Priestman

Coping with Childhood Allergies
Jill Eckersley

Coping with Childhood Asthma
Jill Eckersley

Coping with Chronic Fatigue
Trudie Chalder

Coping with Coeliac Disease
Karen Brody

Coping with Cystitis
Caroline Clayton

Coping with Depression and Elation
Patrick McKeon

Coping with Down's Syndrome
Fiona Marshall

Coping with Dyspraxia
Jill Eckersley

Coping with Eating Disorders and Body Image
Christine Craggs-Hinton

Coping with Eczema
Dr Robert Youngson

Coping with Endometriosis
Jo Mears

Coping with Epilepsy
Fiona Marshall and
Dr Pamela Crawford

Coping with Fibroids
Mary-Claire Mason

Coping with Gout
Christine Craggs-Hinton

Coping with Heartburn and Reflux
Dr Tom Smith

Coping with Incontinence
Dr Joan Gomez

Coping with Long-Term Illness
Barbara Baker

Coping with Macular Degeneration
Dr Patricia Gilbert

Coping with the Menopause
Janet Horwood

Overcoming Common Problems Series

Coping with a Mid-life Crisis
Derek Milne

Coping with Polycystic Ovary Syndrome
Christine Craggs-Hinton

Coping with Postnatal Depression
Sandra L. Wheatley

Coping with SAD
Fiona Marshall and Peter Cheevers

Coping with Snoring and Sleep Apnoea
Jill Eckersley

Coping with a Stressed Nervous System
Dr Kenneth Hambly and Alice Muir

Coping with Strokes
Dr Tom Smith

Coping with Suicide
Maggie Helen

Coping with Thyroid Problems
Dr Joan Gomez

Depression
Dr Paul Hauck

Depression at Work
Vicky Maud

Depressive Illness
Dr Tim Cantopher

Eating for a Healthy Heart
Robert Povey, Jacqui Morrell and Rachel Povey

Effortless Exercise
Dr Caroline Shreeve

Fertility
Julie Reid

Free Your Life from Fear
Jenny Hare

Getting a Good Night's Sleep
Fiona Johnston

Heal the Hurt: How to Forgive and Move On
Dr Ann Macaskill

Heart Attacks – Prevent and Survive
Dr Tom Smith

Help Your Child Get Fit Not Fat
Jan Hurst and Sue Hubberstey

Helping Children Cope with Anxiety
Jill Eckersley

Helping Children Cope with Change and Loss
Rosemary Wells

Helping Children Get the Most from School
Sarah Lawson

How to Be Your Own Best Friend
Dr Paul Hauck

How to Beat Pain
Christine Craggs-Hinton

How to Cope with Bulimia
Dr Joan Gomez

How to Cope with Difficult People
Alan Houel and Christian Godefroy

How to Improve Your Confidence
Dr Kenneth Hambly

How to Keep Your Cholesterol in Check
Dr Robert Povey

How to Stick to a Diet
Deborah Steinberg and Dr Windy Dryden

How to Stop Worrying
Dr Frank Tallis

Hysterectomy
Suzie Hayman

Is HRT Right for You?
Dr Anne MacGregor

Letting Go of Anxiety and Depression
Dr Windy Dryden

Lifting Depression the Balanced Way
Dr Lindsay Corrie

Living with Alzheimer's Disease
Dr Tom Smith

Living with Asperger Syndrome
Dr Joan Gomez

Living with Asthma
Dr Robert Youngson

Living with Autism
Fiona Marshall

Living with Crohn's Disease
Dr Joan Gomez

Living with Diabetes
Dr Joan Gomez

Living with Fibromyalgia
Christine Craggs-Hinton

Living with Food Intolerance
Alex Gazzola

Living with Grief
Dr Tony Lake

Living with Heart Disease
Victor Marks, Dr Monica Lewis and Dr Gerald Lewis

Overcoming Common Problems Series

Living with High Blood Pressure
Dr Tom Smith

Living with Hughes Syndrome
Triona Holden

Living with Loss and Grief
Julia Tugendhat

Living with Lupus
Philippa Pigache

Living with Nut Allergies
Karen Evennett

Living with Osteoarthritis
Dr Patricia Gilbert

Living with Osteoporosis
Dr Joan Gomez

Living with Rheumatoid Arthritis
Philippa Pigache

Living with Sjögren's Syndrome
Sue Dyson

Losing a Baby
Sarah Ewing

Losing a Child
Linda Hurcombe

Make Up or Break Up: Making the Most of Your Marriage
Mary Williams

Making Friends with Your Stepchildren
Rosemary Wells

Making Relationships Work
Alison Waines

Overcoming Anger
Dr Windy Dryden

Overcoming Anxiety
Dr Windy Dryden

Overcoming Back Pain
Dr Tom Smith

Overcoming Depression
Dr Windy Dryden and Sarah Opie

Overcoming Impotence
Mary Williams

Overcoming Jealousy
Dr Windy Dryden

Overcoming Loneliness and Making Friends
Márianna Csóti

Overcoming Procrastination
Dr Windy Dryden

Overcoming Shame
Dr Windy Dryden

Rheumatoid Arthritis
Mary-Claire Mason and Dr Elaine Smith

Shift Your Thinking, Change Your Life
Mo Shapiro

Stress at Work
Mary Hartley

Ten Steps to Positive Living
Dr Windy Dryden

The Assertiveness Handbook
Mary Hartley

The Candida Diet Book
Karen Brody

The Chronic Fatigue Healing Diet
Christine Craggs-Hinton

The Fibromyalgia Healing Diet
Christine Craggs-Hinton

The Irritable Bowel Diet Book
Rosemary Nicol

The PMS Diet Book
Karen Evennett

The Self-Esteem Journal
Alison Waines

The Traveller's Good Health Guide
Ted Lankester

Think Your Way to Happiness
Dr Windy Dryden and Jack Gordon

Treating Arthritis Diet Book
Margaret Hills

Treating Arthritis Exercise Book
Margaret Hills and Janet Horwood

Treating Arthritis – The Drug-Free Way
Margaret Hills

Treating Arthritis – More Ways to a Drug-Free Life
Margaret Hills

Understanding Obsessions and Compulsions
Dr Frank Tallis

When Someone You Love Has Depression
Barbara Baker

Your Man's Health
Fiona Marshall

Overcoming Common Problems

Every Woman's Guide to Heart Health

Jill Eckersley

sheldon**PRESS**

First published in Great Britain in 2006

Sheldon Press
36 Causton Street
London SW1P 4ST

Copyright © Jill Eckersley 2006

The author and publisher have made every effort to ensure that
the external website and email addresses included in this book are
correct and up to date at the time of going to press. The author
and publisher are not responsible for the content, quality or
continuing accessibility of the sites.

British Library Cataloguing-in-Publication Data

A catalogue record for this book is available from the British Library

ISBN-13: 978–0–85969–978–5
ISBN-10: 0–85969–978–1

1 3 5 7 9 10 8 6 4 2

Typeset by Deltatype Limited, Birkenhead, Merseyside
Printed in Great Britain by Ashford Colour Press

Contents

Acknowledgements viii

Introduction ix

1 Know your heart 1

2 When things go wrong 4

3 Maintaining a healthy heart 16

4 Smoking 23

5 Eating for a healthy heart 33

6 Exercise and your heart 42

7 Hormones 51

8 Diabetes 59

9 Stress and high blood pressure 65

10 Living with heart disease 75

11 Heart surgery and rehabilitation 84

Useful addresses and further reading 95

Index 101

Acknowledgements

Thanks to the many people who have helped me with the research for this book. I would especially like to thank the British Heart Foundation, the experts in the field! Many thanks, also, to consultant cardiologist Ghada Mikhail for sparing the time to talk to me, also to the ever-helpful advisers at Heart UK, the Blood Pressure Association and GUCH – the Grown Up Congenital Heart Patients Association. Contact details for these organizations are on pages 95–7.

Special thanks are due to all the heart patients, ex-smokers and others who provided case histories to reassure other women that it's not only possible to prevent heart disease, but also to survive it!

Introduction

Think of a prime candidate for a heart attack, and the chances are the image that springs to mind is an overweight middle-aged executive, with a brandy in one hand and a cigar in the other. And he'll be male. For years, heart disease has been thought of as a man's problem. Research by the British Heart Foundation (BHF) in 2002 discovered that most women think of cancer – and especially breast cancer – as the biggest threat to their health. Young women, in particular the 18–34 age group, are most likely to identify breast and lung cancer as the biggest health threats they face.

The facts are quite different. In 2003, 51,495 women died of coronary heart disease (CHD) in the UK, compared with 13,628 who died from lung cancer and 12,625 who died from breast cancer. CHD is the single biggest killer of women in the UK, with one in six likely to die from it. The BHF has been concerned about women's lack of awareness of heart disease for some time. There are also some studies that suggest that women don't get equal access to investigations and treatment for heart problems, perhaps because even the medical profession still thinks of heart disease as something that happens to men.

The good news is that rates of heart disease are falling, for both men and women. Since the late 1970s, death rates from coronary heart disease have fallen all over the developed world. For people under 65 in the UK, death rates have fallen by an impressive 44 per cent in the last ten years. Medical and surgical treatments for heart disease are improving all the time, with more effective drugs and better surgical techniques. However it's estimated that more than half of the reduction in mortality rates in the 1980s and 1990s was due to lifestyle changes like giving up smoking and eating healthier diets. In other words, there is a great deal we can all do to help ourselves to *prevent* heart disease and *survive* into healthy old age – which is what this book is about!

The not-so-good news is that although death rates are falling, Britain isn't doing as well as some other countries in reducing the amount of CHD among the population. The UK is about halfway up the international table and although the death rate among British women fell by 44 per cent between 1990 and 2000, Australian and New Zealand women saw their death rates fall by 51 per cent and 48 per cent during the same period.

The Government, which has set a target of reducing death rates by two-fifths by 2010, is concerned about certain trends among British women. Smoking is one of the biggest risk factors for heart disease and girls are more likely to be regular smokers than boys, with 10 per cent of 11–15-year-old girls admitting to lighting up. Obesity is another risk factor and too many women in the UK are piling on the pounds. Levels of obesity in this country have *tripled* since 1980 and about half of British women are either overweight or obese.

Then there's the question of exercise. The message is simple: if you want to have a healthy heart, you need to keep moving. Yet according to studies, around four out of ten women don't even have one 30-minute period of exercise a week, when the BHF recommends a minimum of 30 minutes a day.

Not convinced yet that you need to look after your heart? Perhaps you're one of those people who think that heart disease just means a quick death from a sudden heart attack. This isn't so. Living with heart disease can mean years of pain and breathlessness.

But it doesn't have to be that way. The risk factors for heart disease – in women as well as men – are very well known. Some, like old age, or a family history of heart problems, you can't do much about. It's a fact, though, that some very simple lifestyle changes, plus *awareness* of your heart and its welfare, can make all the difference. Heart health isn't just for men – it's for you too!

1

Know your heart

The importance of the heart has been recognized from ancient times, since long before people knew much about the way it worked. The heart has always been considered the seat of the emotions, especially of love. Think of all the expressions we use which include the word 'heart'. We can have a change of heart, live in the heart of the country, break someone's heart, eat our hearts out, set our hearts on something, have our hearts in our mouths, or in the right place. We can be hearty types, we can be heart-throbs, we can have a heart-to-heart or tug someone's heartstrings. No other organ in the body plays such a big part in our day-to-day vocabulary, reflecting the importance of the heart to our health and well-being.

CHD: A modern disease?

Some experts have said that coronary heart disease is very much a twentieth and twenty-first century problem. Heart attacks, they say, were rare before 1900. This may be partly because most of our ancestors didn't live long enough to develop coronary heart disease. Life expectancy in 1900 was only about 50 years, compared with almost 80 years now. However, everyone does agree that heart disease has become the Number One killer in the Western world. It certainly seems that the way we have been living in the last hundred years has led to more and more of us developing heart problems. The World Health Organization described coronary heart disease as 'an epidemic' as long ago as 1940. Between 1948 and 1978 the Framingham Study in the USA identified the causes of this epidemic – smoking, lack of exercise, and poor diet among them. Whereas our ancestors walked or rode, we jump in our cars. Whereas they ate plain, locally produced food, we eat too many highly processed, fatty and sugary treats like burgers, chips and doughnuts. Fewer of us earn our livings doing hard manual labour any more. Housework no longer involves scrubbing and wringing out the washing, beating carpets and churning butter.

The development of heart surgery

William Harvey described the circulation of the blood as long ago as 1628, and by the early eighteenth century, the structure of the heart had been discovered. René Laënnec invented the stethoscope in 1816 so that physicians could hear the human heartbeat. An electrocardiograph was developed in 1903, hardening of the arteries was first described in 1912, and the first heart surgery took place in the USA in 1938. Open-heart surgery was pioneered in 1952. Cardiac massage was first used to re-start a heart in 1961, and in 1967 South African surgeon Christiaan Barnard performed the first ever heart transplant. Today, heart surgery is virtually routine. Just under 30,000 coronary artery bypass operations take place in the UK every year – an increase of one-third over the last decade – and 128 heart transplants were carried out in 2002/2003. There are also around 45,000 coronary angioplasty operations – where the fatty tissue blocking the arteries is 'squashed' by a device, called a 'stent', which holds open the narrowed blood vessel. New drugs, and better combinations of drugs, are coming onto the market all the time.

'Treatments for heart disease are moving ahead at speed,' says the consultant cardiologist, Ghada Mikhail, from the North West London Hospitals and St Mary's Hospital Trust.

> Stent technology is improving, with stents coated with special drugs which reduce the narrowing of the arteries. New surgical techniques include minimally invasive surgery, where the wound is smaller than usual, and off-pump bypass surgery, where the heart continues to beat and a heart–lung bypass machine is not used. There are indications that this type of surgery might benefit women in particular.

The still-controversial stem cell research might, in the future, enable new heart muscle to be 'grown' to replace dead or damaged heart muscle.

Understanding your heart

A normal, healthy heart is about the size of a clenched fist and works like a pump, pumping blood to every single muscle and organ in your body, including the brain, digestive organs, kidneys and skin. It keeps working 24 hours a day, seven days a week, 52 weeks a year. It beats 100,000 times in every 24-hour period, which adds up to 36 million heartbeats in a year. By the time you reach the age of 75, your heart will have beaten 2.74 billion times. It pumps between 5 and 20 litres of blood around your body every minute, depending on whether you are active or resting.

The heart has four chambers. The two upper ones are called the left atrium and the right atrium, and the two lower chambers are called the left and right ventricles. The two atria are 'filling' chambers, which receive the blood; the two ventricles are the 'pumping' chambers, which pump it round again. The left ventricle pumps oxygenated blood to the body; the right ventricle pumps de-oxygenated blood to the lungs, where it becomes oxygenated. The blood is kept flowing in the right direction by valves at the entrances to and exits from each chamber. Like all the body's organs, the heart needs a supply of blood and oxygen to function properly.

Arteries

The blood vessels which carry blood to your heart are called coronary arteries. There are two of them, the left and the right coronary artery. The left coronary artery has two large branches whereas the right coronary artery is one big blood vessel. Coronary arteries are about the size of a drinking straw, 3 to 4 millimetres across, with men's arteries being slightly wider than women's. They have to be quite tough and elastic to cope with the continuous pumping action of the heart and the blood circulating within them, right down to the narrow vessels which feed the inner layers of the heart muscle.

Veins

Veins – which you can often see on the back of your hands or legs – have thinner walls than arteries and often look blue. They carry de-oxygenated blood back to the heart after the oxygen and nutrients it contains have been used up by the other organs of the body.

3

2

When things go wrong

Some people are born with heart problems, including inherited conditions like cardiomyopathy (see pages 10–13) or faulty heart valves. Others develop heart disease later in life.

Atherosclerosis and heart attack

Deaths from heart disease are the result of atherosclerosis – the clogging up of the blood vessels by fatty deposits, like sludge in a pipe. Healthy arteries have a smooth lining called the endothelium, past which blood can flow quite freely. As the arteries narrow, it becomes more and more difficult for the blood to flow and for the heart muscle to obtain the blood and oxygen it needs. Eventually a blood clot may form, blocking the artery completely and cutting off the blood supply, causing a heart attack. A heart attack is sometimes called a coronary or a myocardial infarction (MI). About 117,500 women in the UK have a heart attack every year, compared with about 142,000 men.

Symptoms of a heart attack
These include:

- chest pain – especially if it is not connected to exertion, and lasts more than a few moments. It can be a crushing pain, a feeling of uncomfortable pressure, fullness or squeezing, or as though there is a tight band around the chest;
- pain that spreads to the shoulders, neck or arms, upper abdomen or jaw;
- chest pain accompanied by light-headedness, fainting, sweating, nausea, vomiting or breathlessness;
- anxiety, nervousness;
- pale, sweaty skin.

Some heart attacks are 'silent' and don't cause excessive pain, so that sufferers may not even be aware that they have had a heart attack at all. A study based on more than 4,000 Dutch people, and reported in the *European Heart Journal* in early 2006, found that about four in ten heart attacks are not recognized at the time. Cardiologist Ghada Mikhail, writing in the British Medical Journal in 2005, pointed out that women's symptoms are often less obvious than men's and can include a burning feeling in the chest, abdominal discomfort and fatigue, as well as more typical symptoms. The Dutch study confirmed this with fewer than half of the women recognizing a heart attack for what it was. Chest pain and breathlessness, especially if the pain is severe, lasts longer than a few minutes, and doesn't respond to ordinary indigestion remedies, should be reported to your GP or NHS Direct.

What to do for a suspected heart attack
If you suspect a heart attack:

- dial 999 and ask for an ambulance, explaining that you think the person has had a heart attack, as a specially equipped ambulance will be sent;
- lie the person down with her head and shoulders supported by pillows, cushions, a coat – whatever is available – so that she is in a semi-sitting position. Loosen any tight clothing and reassure the person that help is on the way;
- remember that more than half of those who have a heart attack survive because of prompt medical attention. Someone who receives the right drugs within an hour of having a heart attack has a much reduced risk of long-term damage to the heart.

Lorna
Lorna was in her late fifties when she began having symptoms. 'I didn't associate them with heart problems,' she says.

> I had had high blood pressure for some time and had to take tablets, and was also taking cholesterol-lowering drugs. When I started to have shooting pains, they seemed to be more in my stomach than my chest, and I took no notice. Then we went on a family outing on a very hot day and I began to feel ill and breathless. I took time off work, as my job was quite stressful, and then awoke one night with a knife-like pain in my chest. I really felt as though someone had thrust a knife through me

5

and was twisting it. I also felt sick. It did occur to me that it could be a heart attack but I didn't really believe it was. My husband insisted I went to our GP, who told me I should be in hospital.

Looking back, I still find it hard to believe that I managed to walk from the car park into A&E, where the doctors put me on a trolley, did some blood tests and told me I had had a heart attack!

Bridget
Bridget was only 44 when she had her heart attack. Like Lorna, she didn't think she was at risk. 'I was a smoker, though I had planned to give up before I hit the menopause,' she says.

With a full-time job and two children, I was often stressed, but when I complained to my GP of pains at the top right-hand side of my stomach, he prescribed antacids. I wondered if I could have gallstones as the pain was sharp enough to take my breath away. It was there whether I rested or walked about. Eventually, as the pain seemed to be getting worse, I called an ambulance. I don't think even the paramedic thought I was having a heart attack as I was so young, though he did give me aspirin. The hospital gave me an ECG [electrocardiogram] and trolleyed me into Resus, where my condition was stabilized. Within 24 hours, I was in a specialized coronary care unit and had been prescribed a cocktail of heart drugs.

I couldn't believe it when they told me what was wrong. It was truly a life-changing moment. My father had a heart attack at 51 and is still alive today but I never thought it would happen to me.

Angina

Not all chest pains mean that you are having a heart attack. The British Heart Foundation estimates that there are about 840,000 women in the UK who have, or have had, angina. Angina can cause chest pain and breathlessness when you exert yourself, for example running for a bus, or when you become very angry, over-stressed or excited. It's a symptom, rather than a disease in itself, and occurs because your arteries are 'furring up' like blocked pipes. They are becoming narrower, too narrow for the right amount of blood and oxygen to reach the heart muscle.

Unlike the pain of a heart attack, pain caused by angina usually goes within 10 or 15 minutes if you rest and relax. It's sometimes hard to tell the difference, especially if this is the first time you have experienced chest pain, or any pain that radiates to your neck, arm, jaw, and even your back or stomach. Angina pain can:

- feel like a burning, tight feeling in your chest;
- make it difficult for you to breathe;
- be felt in other areas of your body in addition to, or instead of your chest – for example your back or your stomach;
- usually be linked to extra effort – perhaps walking uphill or carrying something heavy;
- come on if you are upset, stressed or angry, or in specially cold weather.

Treatment, in the form of drugs and sprays, is available for angina and it's important that you get a definite diagnosis. 'Stable' angina is when your chest pain comes on after a predictable amount of exercise or stress, and responds well to drugs. 'Unstable' angina is when you have a first episode of chest pain, or when the pain comes on when you are resting or after an unpredictable amount of exercise, or in different circumstances from usual. Never ignore severe chest pains. Make an appointment to see your GP and explain what has happened.

Anna
Anna, 45, was rushed to hospital with chest pains. An angiogram revealed she had three blockages in her arteries and angina was diagnosed.

> In the four years since I was diagnosed I have learned to manage my condition, but it has changed my life . . . I worked as a psychiatric nurse and I had to give up my job. We also moved to a bungalow as I couldn't walk upstairs. I have been given a variety of medication, including what they call a GTN [glyceryl trinitrate] spray which I can use if ever I feel the pain coming on.
> For months I was chair- and bed-bound and could barely

make it to the loo on my own, but slowly my condition has improved. I can go out locally if I'm careful, and I can even drive, though I'm not allowed to carry heavy shopping. It has been very, very hard on my partner, who has had to take over much of the housework and cooking. I have to avoid humid air and steamy atmospheres as well as cold, damp, foggy weather. Stress and emotion can bring on the symptoms too. I always say I've used up at least two of my nine lives, but I plan to enjoy the other seven.

Heart failure

Heart failure means what it says: it's the heart's inability to do its job in pumping the right amount of blood and oxygen around the body. About 404,000 women over 45 in the UK have heart failure. Symptoms of heart failure include:

- breathlessness, which may happen only when you exert yourself, like the pain of angina. In more serious cases you may become so short of breath that you can only walk with difficulty, and feel breathless even when sitting or lying down. Breathlessness is one of the earliest signs of heart failure and can build up over weeks or months;
- fluid retention, which can cause your ankles and lower legs to swell up and, if left untreated, can lead to swelling of your abdomen as well;
- fatigue, because your heart is unable to pump the blood round your body efficiently and your body does not receive the nutrients it needs.

Like angina, heart failure can be managed with a combination of drug treatments and lifestyle changes.

Sally
Sally was a fit, 36-year-old mum of three small children with no family history of heart problems when she had her first heart attack. She was eventually diagnosed with an extremely rare condition called spontaneous coronary artery dissection, leading to heart failure. Her husband was told there was nothing doctors could do for her.

I was at a children's party when I collapsed with dreadful chest pains. At first I was diagnosed with indigestion but when it happened again four days later, hospital tests revealed I had had a heart attack.

I was transferred to a coronary care unit where I had another attack and that was the point when I realized I was fighting for my life. Strangely enough, I wasn't terrified, I just knew I had to keep breathing. It was a bit like being in labour, instinct took over and I hung on . . .

Hours passed, then days. I had no energy to speak or even blink, but somehow enough blood and oxygen seemed to find its way through my damaged arteries to keep me alive. I've been told that once you have heart failure, the heart can't repair itself, but mine seems to have done so even though it's damaged. I can see the dead muscle when I have a scan, but my heart does seem to be doing its job.

I'm on a cocktail of drugs and have to have regular blood tests to check for liver or kidney damage. After eighteen months I was leading a normal life and thinking about going back to work. It has been an emotional, as well as a physical battle. I grieved for the loss of my health, I get tired easily, and I worry about catching something like flu in case I end up in hospital. But I try to think positive and am involved with heart rehabilitation groups. It's rather like living with a ticking time bomb!

Heart disease

Some forms of heart disease are concerned with disturbances of the heart rhythm – or arrhythmia, or conditions which affect the actual muscle of the heart, rather than its blood flow – such as cardiomyopathy.

Arrhythmia

Arrhythmia simply means an irregular or abnormal heartbeat, which can cause symptoms such as light-headedness, fainting, dizziness and palpitations. The heart may be beating too fast – tachycardia, or too slowly – bradycardia. The heart has its own natural pacemaker (a small amount of nerve tissue in the right atrium) that ensures that the heart beats with a steady, regular rhythm. Minor disturbances of this rhythm, which may be caused by, for example, drinking too much strong coffee, are nothing to worry about. Arrhythmia can also be caused by a birth defect, coronary heart disease, or an over-active thyroid gland. Some drugs can also have this effect.

Arrhythmia may affect the upper chambers of the heart, the atria, in which case it is known as atrial fibrillation. It can also affect the lower chambers or ventricles, and can sometimes cause a condition known as heart block in which the normal electrical impulses that stimulate the heartbeat are interrupted, causing breathlessness, fainting and blackouts. Arrhythmia can be treated with drugs or by having an artificial heart pacemaker fitted.

Jenny

Jenny, 49, has recently had a pacemaker fitted.

> About a year ago I started to have palpitations and went to my GP. Atrial fibrillation was diagnosed, and I was offered drugs to help. Unfortunately the symptoms continued and I began to feel faint and breathless, so I was admitted to my local hospital to have a pacemaker fitted.
>
> The operation took place under local anaesthetic. A small incision was made at the top of my chest to insert the pacemaker which is tiny – smaller than a matchbox. I was in hospital for a couple of days and it wasn't really painful, only a bit uncomfortable. I was told that it will have to be changed in maybe six to ten years.
>
> I got used to it surprisingly quickly. I try to look after my health anyway, but I'm specially careful to eat well and do moderate exercise. I get the occasional attack of palpitations, but feel fine most of the time!

Cardiomyopathy

Cardiomyopathy is a condition – in fact, a number of conditions – in which the heart muscle is abnormal in some way, which prevents it from working properly. There are four different types:

- Hypertrophic cardiomyopathy (HCM)
- Dilated cardiomyopathy (DCM)
- Arrhythmogenic Right Ventricular Cardiomyopathy (ARVC)
- Restrictive cardiomyopathy.

Hypertrophic Cardiomyopathy is by far the most common, affecting perhaps 1 in 500 people in the UK.

As yet, we do not know what causes cardiomyopathy, but it is an inherited disorder, transmitted from one generation to the next. The children of someone affected by hypertrophic cardiomyopathy have a 50:50 chance of inheriting the condition. Once a patient has been diagnosed, the rest of the family will need to be screened for the condition.

Hypertrophy literally means 'to thicken', and the main feature of this kind of cardiomyopathy is thickening of the heart muscle. Children may be born with hypertrophic cardiomyopathy but it doesn't usually become evident until adolescence or young adulthood. Some people, however, do develop it in later life. Symptoms include breathlessness, fatigue, chest pain, light-headedness, fainting or blackouts, sometimes after exercise.

Stephanie
Stephanie was a 26-year-old nurse and mother of a two-year-old son when she blacked out on the treadmill at her local gym.

They managed to resuscitate me and called an ambulance but I had ten more cardiac arrests that day and spent 48 hours on life support. My family were told I only had a 10 per cent chance of pulling through.

A few days later the consultant told me I had hypertrophic cardiomyopathy. Even though I am a nurse I had never heard of it. My first thought was *what, me?* I had never had any symptoms apart from occasional palpitations. When I learned more about it I was terrified of dropping dead and worried that I had passed it on to my son.

I was originally prescribed a drug called amiodarone, and then in 1995 I had an ICD (an implantable cardioverter defibrillator – a device similar to a pacemaker) fitted. It has changed my life! I can run, play tennis, swim, travel and lead a normal life. I now work with cardio patients and can tell them, honestly, that life does go on. Some people need no treatment, others need surgery, and treatments are improving all the time. I used to be a smoker but have given up, I watch my weight and eat a healthy diet. When I was first diagnosed, I thought life was over for me but since then I have completed an MA

11

and had another baby. Luckily, neither of my sons has inherited the condition.

Jacqui

Jacqui, 36, was eight months pregnant when she developed dilated cardiomyopathy, a condition in which the heart becomes enlarged and is able to pump less strongly.

To be honest I don't remember much about it. I became very breathless and thought I had a chest infection. My husband was so worried he called out the emergency doctor and I was rushed to hospital. I can remember being given oxygen in hospital . . . and woke up three weeks later in cardiac intensive care. My son was born by emergency Caesarian. I didn't even see him until he was three weeks old.

I didn't grasp how ill I was though I do remember a consultant saying that if I didn't improve my only hope would be a transplant.

However my heart seemed to respond to all the drugs I was given. I was on 14 different tablets a day at one point. I had regular check-ups and scans, and gradually learned to walk again as well as looking after my baby. Six months later I was told my heart was back to normal and now, two-and-a-half years later, I lead a normal life. It took ages for my confidence to come back. I have been advised to have no more children as the condition could develop again in another pregnancy. I'm lucky to have my son and lucky to be alive!

Eve

Eve, 43, was aware there were heart problems in her family. Her sister had collapsed and died after playing squash, when she was in her 20s.

I kept getting palpitations and eventually went to hospital for a check-up where I was given an ECG and an echocardiogram. I was referred to the London Heart Hospital where I was told I had ARVC, which causes abnormal electrical heart rhythms.

At first I felt as though I had a guillotine hanging over my head as I was aware I could just keel over and die. I was prescribed anti-arrhythmia drugs and then, a year later, I was given an ICD – an implantable cardioverter defibrillator. It 'paces' my heart rhythms, or gives me a shock if I need one. It felt strange at first but I'm used to it now.

I can only work part-time as I get rather tired, and I can no longer play sport, which I loved, but other than that my life is pretty normal. The main thing I worry about is whether I have passed the condition on to my son, who is being carefully monitored.

The Cardiomyopathy Association (contact details on page 96) is a voluntary organization which supports those with cardiomyopathy and their families.

Familial hypercholesterolaemia

More than 100,000 people in Britain have another inherited condition, familial hypercholesterolaemia (FH), which is caused by an abnormal gene. It leads to exceptionally high levels of cholesterol in the blood. High cholesterol is a well-known risk factor for coronary heart disease. (For more about cholesterol and what it means for heart health, see Chapter 5.) If it remains untreated, CHD can develop in early middle age or sometimes earlier. Risk factors for FH include very high cholesterol and/or a family history of heart disease. Symptoms include 'lumps and bumps' – formed from cholesterol deposits – which sometimes appear on the knuckles and heels and around the eyes.

Treatment for FH includes careful diet management and drug treatment aimed at lowering cholesterol levels.

Familial combined hyperlipidaemia

This is a similar inherited condition in which the amount of triglycerides – fats in the blood – are raised to a dangerous level, as well as cholesterol. Like FH it is associated with early onset CHD and is treated with a combination of healthy diet and lifestyle changes, and a drug regime.

Marfan syndrome

Another inherited disorder which can affect the heart is Marfan syndrome. It affects about 10,000 people in this country, 1 in 10 of whom are estimated to have heart problems. It's caused by an abnormal gene, identified in 1990, which affects the production of fibrillin, a fine fibre found the body's connective tissues. Marfan patients can have weakened and more fragile blood vessels in their hearts and/or problems with the heart valves, leading to irregular heart rhythms and sometimes heart failure. The condition needs to be carefully monitored. It can be treated with drugs like beta-blockers and sometimes heart surgery. There is a Marfan Association (contact details on pages 97–8) which offers advice and support to patients and families.

Valvular heart disease

There are four valves in the heart, at the entrances and exits to each of the four chambers. Their job is to make sure that the blood flows in the right direction. Some people are born with faulty heart valves; others develop problems later in life, either as a result of the ageing process or as a long-term effect of disease like rheumatic fever (though this is now much less common in Britain than it used to be.)

There are two kinds of valve problems. One, called 'stenosis', means the valve isn't opening properly and blood flow is impeded. The other, called 'incompetence', means that the valve isn't closing completely, and blood is leaking backwards. In both cases, the heart has to work harder and this puts a strain on it.

Some people with valvular heart disease have few symptoms; others suffer from breathlessness, palpitations, swollen ankles or legs, and sometimes chest pain. Treatment can include drugs and, if necessary, replacement valve surgery.

Endocarditis

This is an infection of the lining of the heart or the heart valves. Healthy hearts can become infected, but the disease is most likely to attack those who are already vulnerable through heart abnormalities, old age, existing illness or a weakened immune system – for instance, after heart surgery. Endocarditis is usually caused by a bacterium, more rarely by a virus or fungus. One of the most common causes of infection is dental treatment, as bacteria in the mouth can easily get into the bloodstream if the gums bleed during dental procedures. Good dental hygiene is important for everyone, and heart patients will be given advice on procedures to follow when they visit the dentist. Normally, antibiotics should be taken before treatment.

Symptoms include fever, night sweats, a general feeling of illness, weight loss and – if it remains untreated – heart failure, stroke and kidney damage. Diagnosis is by echocardiogram and blood tests and treatment is with antibiotics.

Living with a congenital heart defect

Congenital heart defects are often picked up during the mother's pregnancy or shortly after birth. Since the 1960s, open-heart surgery has been performed on children, so a whole generation of people have grown up after surviving heart problems which might have killed them in the past. Most women who have grown up with congenital heart defects lead normal lives. Some have to take medication, some have to have regular check-ups with a cardiologist. There is a support group called GUCH (the Grown Up Congenital Heart Patients Association) which gives information and advice. Contact details are on page 97.

3

Maintaining a healthy heart

Raising awareness

Even thinking about the possibility of heart disease can be alarming and the idea of having 'heart trouble' can be stressful in itself. But it's not all bad news. First of all, treatments for heart problems are advancing all the time. Conditions which would have meant a premature death just a few years ago are now treatable with drugs and/or surgery. Research is ongoing into the genetic factors which influence which of us develop heart problems and, in time, it may be possible to screen those most at risk.

It's also true that much more is known about the risk factors for heart disease and many of these are avoidable. For most of us, heart health is in our own hands, so to speak! The Government has set a target of reducing the death rate from heart disease by 40 per cent by the year 2010, and there are signs that this target will be met. The chances of this happening are greater if we all make a few simple lifestyle changes. This is already beginning to happen as many of us become more aware of healthy eating, the importance of exercise, and how vital it is to give up smoking. We shall be looking at these factors in greater detail in later chapters.

The medical profession and organizations like the British Heart Foundation are also trying hard to raise awareness of the risks of heart disease in women, who have been neglected in the past as coronary heart disease was thought of as a 'man's problem'.

'Historically, women have tended to be under-diagnosed, under-treated and under-researched,' says cardiologist Ghada Mikhail.

There is also concern that some women are not modifying their risk factors. It's true that heart disease is much more common in older, post-menopausal women, but arteries can start to fur up from the age of 20! It's really important for all women to pay attention to factors like healthy diets, giving up smoking, and being aware of their blood pressure and cholesterol levels.

There are some special problems for women. They can find it harder to give up smoking than men do. Diabetic women are at greater risk of heart problems than diabetic men.

16

Women also tend to have less 'typical' symptoms of heart attacks. While a man might have the typical crushing chest pain, a woman might have abdominal, shoulder or jaw pain and simply not consider the idea of a heart attack. So women tend to go to their GP or A&E rather later. As with any illness, the sooner you are diagnosed the better the outcome. At the moment, women who have an angioplasty or bypass surgery tend not to do as well as men. Their blood vessels are smaller and more difficult to treat, and because they are having treatment later they may have more complicating factors like high blood pressure, high cholesterol or diabetes. Most drug trials are also carried out on men.

Recently, both the American Heart Association and the European Society of Cardiology have been starting to redress the balance so that better guidelines on heart care for women can be put together. In the meantime, there's a lot we can do to help ourselves.

Risk factors

Family history

Of course there are some risk factors that individuals can't do much about. Family history matters. The BHF says that if you have one or more close blood relatives – mother, father, sisters or brothers – who have developed angina or had a heart attack before the age of 55, for men, and 65, for women, you need to be specially careful, and should tell your GP and/or practice nurse. It might be that there is an inherited tendency for high blood pressure or high cholesterol – both well-known risk factors for heart disease – in your family. Your GP will be able to test both your cholesterol levels and your blood pressure to make sure that all is well. (For more information about the importance of cholesterol, see Chapter 5, and for more information about blood pressure, see Chapter 9.) Whatever your family history, a combination of sensible lifestyle changes and possibly medication, if you need it, can control both blood pressure and cholesterol levels.

Age

Age is another risk factor – more people have heart problems in their seventies than in their thirties, and none of us can help getting older! But, however young or old you are, you can still look after your heart.

The example of Finland

We could all learn lessons from what has happened in Finland. In the 1970s, Finland topped the 'World's Unhealthiest Country' polls, with heart disease at record levels. Most people smoked, ate a lot of full-fat dairy products, and didn't take much exercise.

'Finnish men used to say that vegetables were for rabbits, not real men, so people simply did not eat vegetables,' says the country's director of public health. The Government made a real effort to convince people to change their way of life, with the result that life expectancy for Finnish women is now six years longer than it was before the lifestyle-changing measures were brought in. These measures included:

- a complete ban on tobacco advertising; plus local 'quit-smoking' competitions with prizes;
- local cholesterol-lowering competitions with prizes;
- a drive to produce low-fat milk on the country's farms;
- incentives for growers to produce more local fruit like berries;
- cheap, clean local sports facilities like swimming pools, ball parks and snow parks;
- well-maintained and well-lit walking and cycle paths.

If the Finns can do it, why can't we? The trouble is that getting fit and staying healthy is so often presented as something we *ought* to do, rather than something we *want* to do. Looking after your heart shouldn't be a matter of giving up this and denying yourself that. You can still enjoy life – in fact, when you're healthy, you enjoy life *more*. You sleep better, you're ready to face the day instead of crawling out of bed in the morning desperate for your 'fix' of caffeine to get you through. You don't have to become a gym fanatic or give up life's little pleasures like the occasional doughnut, glass of good wine or a chocolate bar. If you are a 20-a-day smoker, when you do manage to ditch those cigarettes you could find yourself with as much as £1,700 a year to spend on a holiday in the sun or a couple of breaks at a health farm being pampered. Not convinced yet? Let's take a look at the risk factors and ways to avoid them.

The risk factors

Smoking

Smoking is one of the most important risk factors for CHD, as well as lung cancer and most other killer diseases. It's been estimated that about half of all regular smokers will die prematurely because of their habit. That doesn't just mean the possibility of a quick death from a heart attack, but months, possibly years of debilitating illness. Only about a quarter of British women are now smokers, and most of them probably want to give up, for health or financial reasons. Most women now know that smoking harms them, their children, and also their unborn babies. Only 20 per cent of pregnant women now smoke and the Government is hoping that this figure will fall to 15 per cent by 2010. Banning smoking in all enclosed public spaces from the summer of 2007 can only help. Inhaling second-hand smoke (so-called 'passive smoking') increases the risk of CHD by 25 per cent.

There's still some concern about the number of young teenage girls who smoke. As anyone who had tried it knows, giving up can be tough, and it's so much easier not to start. One in ten girls aged under 15 claims to be a regular smoker.

Eating the wrong food

Diet is a tremendously important factor in the development of heart disease. In Britain, as in most of the affluent West, we're no longer dying of the infectious diseases that carried off so many in the past. Instead, we are dying of over-consumption; which means that we are tending to eat the wrong things. Put simply, we are eating too much saturated fat, too much sugar and too much salt, and not enough complex carbohydrates, fruit and vegetables. We all know how hard it is getting children to eat their greens, and health surveys suggest that only just over one in ten children are getting their recommended five portions a day of fruit and veg. Adults don't do much better, with only 15 per cent of women hitting the five-a-day target. The result is that we are all getting fatter. According to the Food Standards Agency, levels of obesity have *tripled* since 1980 and, if present trends continue, this generation of children may die younger than their parents did. Overweight people are at higher risk of CHD. Their hearts have to work so much harder. Imagine carrying a stone of potatoes around with you everywhere and you'll get some idea of the extra strain you are putting on your heart if you are even a stone overweight. Over half the women in Britain are either overweight or obese – which means 30 per cent or more above the right weight for their height.

High cholesterol

High cholesterol levels are also linked with heart disease. Cholesterol is a fatty substance produced naturally by the body and also obtained from the diet, especially from things like eggs, liver and kidneys. Some cholesterol is essential for health but many of us have higher cholesterol than we need. There are two types – LDL or 'bad' cholesterol, which clogs up the arteries, and HDL or 'good' cholesterol, which carries the bad cholesterol away from the arteries and back to the liver. A healthy diet, low in saturated fats, can help to reduce cholesterol levels to below 4.0 mmol.

Lack of exercise

We are just so much less active than we were in the past. Fewer of us are employed in manual jobs. Housework is more a matter of pressing the control panels on the washing machine than scrubbing, wringing and pegging the washing out on the line. It's easy to hop into the car to go to the supermarket . . . or to the cinema, to see friends or out for a meal. Many office workers' opportunity to exercise is limited to a few steps from the front door to the car and a few more from the car park to the office. The Government's recommendation is that we should all do a minimum of 30 minutes of moderate-intensity activity, at least five times a week, to benefit our hearts. Between two-thirds and three-quarters of UK adults do less than that, and about one-third of us don't do any, particularly as we get older. Only 13 per cent of women aged over 65 manage the recommended 30 minutes a day, five times a week. Remember that your heart is a muscle, and like all muscles it will become weak if it isn't efficiently used.

Hormonal change

Before the menopause – which happens to most women between the ages of 45 and 55 – men are more at risk of CHD than women. In 2003, almost four times as many men as women in the 35–44 age group died of heart attacks. It seems that female hormones like oestrogen have a protective effect. When women's periods stop, the levels of oestrogen in their bodies fall and the risk of CHD increases.

Diabetes

People with diabetes are two to four times more likely to suffer from heart disease than the general population, so it's particularly important for diabetics to follow healthy lifestyle guidelines. That means giving up smoking, eating healthily, paying attention to blood pressure and cholesterol levels, getting plenty of exercise and drinking in moderation. The charity Diabetes UK (contact details on page 96) can offer help and advice. They estimate that there are 1.4 million people living with diabetes in the UK, and probably almost as many still un-diagnosed. Diabetes is diagnosed by a simple blood test.

Alcohol

The good news is that moderate alcohol consumption, which means a maximum of a couple of glasses of wine a day, can actually benefit the heart. This only applies to older women, though, whose risk of heart disease after the menopause is greater in any case. It definitely doesn't mean that binge-drinking is good for you – at any age! In fact, drinking more than the recommended maximum for women of 14 units a week is likely to make you put on weight and increase your blood pressure, both of which are risk factors for heart disease. So, where alcohol is concerned, moderation is the key.

High blood pressure

Everyone should have blood pressure checks on a regular basis. High blood pressure is associated with age – fewer than 2 per cent of 16–24 year olds suffer from it, compared with more than half of the over-55s. One study suggested that almost a quarter of all heart attacks are associated with a history of high blood pressure. Blood pressure varies through the day. It goes down when you are asleep and can go up if you are busy or stressed. For most people, blood pressure should be less than 140/90.

Stress

Stress is a much-misunderstood term. We all need some excitement in our lives and some people thrive on it! However, according to the BHF, psycho-social factors like work stress, depression and anxiety,

21

and personality factors like anger and hostility can increase the risk of heart problems. Stress can also be the cause of symptoms like chest pain, breathlessness and panic attacks, which can be confused with heart attacks. Learning to relax and take life more slowly and easily can only benefit heart health.

Periodontal disease

It may sound unlikely but if you don't look after your teeth and gums you could be at greater risk of heart problems. As many as 40 clinical studies have made the link between gum disease and heart disease. As yet, exactly why this happens is not known. It could be because bacteria enter the bloodstream via the inflamed gums and injure the blood vessels, or because the body's own immune response triggers the production of proteins which can damage the arteries.

You can see that there's a lot we can all do to make sure our hearts are as healthy as possible. And it's not all self-sacrifice; there are plenty of pleasurable activities which have been shown to help heart health. A study at Oxford University, published in the journal *Heart*, found that listening to Beethoven's symphonies induced a state of calm which was similar to that induced by beta-blockers. Laughter may indeed be the best medicine. Watching a funny film can help to improve blood flow, according to researchers at the University of Maryland. Chocolate, apples and red wine – in moderation – have also been found to be heart-healthy. Women who have regular sex have higher levels of oestrogen in their blood, leading to a healthier cardiovascular system, lower bad LDL cholesterol and higher good HDL cholesterol. A good night's sleep, walking the dog, and stroking the cat have all been suggested as ways to make sure your heart is in good shape!

4

Smoking

Facts and figures

According to the US Surgeon-General, smoking is 'the most important of the known modifiable risk factors' for coronary heart disease. We know that smoking causes all kinds of other health problems as well, from lung cancer to low-birthweight babies – but did you know that it's now thought that as many as *one in two* smokers will be killed by their habit?

Just under a quarter of British women now smoke and according to health charity ASH, about 80 per cent of those who do have tried to give up at some time. There are still more men (28 per cent) than women (24 per cent) smoking, but there is also concern about the number of young girls who smoke. Maybe because they think it's cool, maybe because they think it will keep their weight down, teenage girls in Britain and elsewhere in the world are continuing to take up smoking.

At the moment, it's estimated that about one in four deaths from heart disease is caused by smoking. The Government's health target is to cut the rate of CHD and stroke by 40 per cent by the year 2010. All local health authorities now have smoking cessation clinics. All NHS buildings will become smoke-free this year, and by the summer of 2007, smoking should be banned in almost all enclosed public places.

Give it up!

If you're a smoker there is really only one way to cut your risk of developing heart disease, and that's by *giving up*. Cutting down on the number of cigarettes you smoke, or switching to low-tar brands, unfortunately doesn't work. Even being a light smoker harms your heart. American researchers found that women who smoked four cigarettes a day had two and a half times the risk of developing CHD or having a heart attack. Danish researchers found that smoking between three and five cigarettes a day led to a significant increase in the risk of heart problems, especially for women. It is also thought that smokers of low-tar cigarettes have to inhale more deeply to get their fix of nicotine, which is not good news for hearts or lungs.

Why is smoking so damaging?

The ingredients in tobacco smoke include nicotine, tar, carbon monoxide and a cocktail of deadly chemicals, any or all of which can damage the body.

Nicotine

This is one of the most addictive substances known, which is why some people find it so difficult to give up smoking. It's a potent poison which is used in insecticides. Nicotine's effect on the body is complex, and includes increasing the heart rate and blood pressure as well as affecting the smoker's mood and behaviour.

Carbon monoxide

Carbon monoxide is a poisonous gas which can kill if it is inhaled in large amounts. High concentrations of carbon monoxide are present in tobacco smoke. Because it dissolves in the blood more quickly than oxygen does, it then attaches itself to the red blood cells, where the oxygen ought to be. It can cut the amount of oxygen in the blood by as much as 15 per cent.

Tar

Tar is the brown gunge which stains a smokers' teeth and fingers yellowish brown. About 70 per cent of the tar in cigarette smoke stays in the smoker's lungs.

Other chemicals

Cigarette smoke also contains acetone, the chemical used in nail varnish remover; ammonia, found in cleaning fluids; the deadly poison arsenic; benzene, which is used as a solvent in fuel; ethanol, the chemical used in anti-freeze; the highly poisonous metal cadmium; formaldehyde, the chemical sometimes used to preserve dead bodies; and the industrial pollutant hydrogen cyanide. Not a very attractive-sounding mixture, is it?

What happens when you smoke

Within one minute of lighting up, your heart rate rises and within ten minutes it may increase by as much as 10 per cent. The nicotine in cigarettes raises your blood pressure and your blood vessels become constricted, so your heart has to work harder. The carbon monoxide in cigarette smoke has a negative effect on your heart as it reduces the blood's ability to carry oxygen around your body.

Smoking increases your cholesterol levels, and the ratio of 'good' (HDL) to 'bad' (LDL) cholesterol is lower in smokers than it is in non-smokers.

Smoking also raises the levels of a protein called fibrinogen in your blood, which makes it stickier and more likely to clot, increasing the risk of a heart attack.

Smokers' arteries have been found to be more rigid and narrower. Narrower arteries, stickier blood and less oxygen all mean that a smoker's heart has to work much harder than a non-smoker's.

What happens when you give up?

This is where the good news starts – and it starts very soon after that last puff!

- Within *20 minutes* your blood pressure and pulse rate will return to normal, and your circulation will improve.
- Within *8 hours* the oxygen levels in your blood increase to a normal level, and your chances of having a heart attack begin to fall.
- Within *24 hours* carbon monoxide leaves your body and your lungs start to clear out mucus and tar (which is why those giving up smoking often get a cough in the first few days).
- Within *48 hours* nicotine can no longer be found in your body and your senses of taste and smell begin to improve.
- Within *72 hours* your energy levels increase and your breathing becomes easier.
- Within *2–12* weeks, your circulation will improve so that walking and exercise all become easier.
- Within *3–9 months* any breathing problems you had will improve.
- Within *5 years* your risk of having a heart attack falls to about half that of a smoker.

- Within *10 years* your risk of a heart attack falls to about the same level as that of someone who has never smoked (and your risk of developing lung cancer falls to around half that of a smoker).

It's worth remembering, too, that even if you have already been diagnosed with heart problems, giving up smoking can increase your chances of a return to good health. If you give up smoking after you have had a heart attack, you effectively *halve* your risk of having another. The British Heart Foundation tells cardiac patients that giving up smoking is the single most important step they can take to aid their recovery. The risk of having another heart attack begins to go down from the moment you stub out your final cigarette.

Passive smoking

This simply means breathing in other people's smoke and yes, it can harm your heart. According to health campaigners ASH, being exposed to high levels of other people's smoke can increase your risk of heart disease by as much as 50 or 60 per cent. One Japanese research study found that as little as 30 minutes of exposure to tobacco smoke can have an impact on blood flow.

If you want to look after your heart, the message is clear: keep away from smoky atmospheres. Ask visitors to your home to smoke outside, or to smoke before they come and see you. If you're driving with smokers, stop for 'smoking breaks' rather than letting them smoke in the confined space of your car. Always choose non-smoking carriages or areas in buses, trains, aircraft, restaurants and all public places. Many are already smoke-free in Britain, and all enclosed public spaces should be smoke-free by 2007.

Finding the motivation to give up

If you're a smoker the chances are you feel a bit guilty about your addiction – and an addiction is what it is. You probably, like roughly eight out of ten women who smoke, would like to give up, but how? Nicotine is horribly addictive and maybe you've tried and failed before. Or maybe you justify it to yourself saying that you have to have *some* vices. There is evidence from America that women do find giving up smoking harder than men do, although British researchers don't necessarily agree.

However, if you're serious about taking care of your heart, the cigarettes have got to go. If the health arguments aren't enough to convince you, what about the other arguments? There's the money, for a start. Think of the whopping £1,700 a year you could save if you gave up your 20-a-day habit, and plan what you'd do with the money. Or, you could ask yourself what smoking is doing to your looks. Teenagers might be able to get away with it, looks-wise (though you could remind your teenage daughter that kissing a smoker is said to be like licking an ashtray), but a study of identical twins found that the non-smoker looked 10 years younger than the smoker by the time they were 40.

You need to be motivated to give up smoking successfully. You might find there's some tiny incident, or some apparently insignificant factor, that finally spurs you into giving up.

'I was struggling with cravings and wondering whether it was worth it. Then I found an old jumper at the back of the wardrobe, took a sniff, and nearly threw up,' says ex-smoker Lesley. 'I couldn't believe I used to go around smelling like that!'

'I finally gave up because smoking was too much hassle,' says Julie, another former smoker. 'I was forever scrabbling around for my fags or my lighter, leaving them in the wrong handbag, worrying if I had enough to last the weekend or having to run down to the corner shop halfway through the evening. I realized how pathetic I was being and that made it easier to give up.'

'I visited my grandad in hospital, on oxygen and hardly able to breathe,' says Lucy. 'He's been a heavy smoker all his life and it was awful seeing him like that. I haven't touched a cigarette since.'

'I had a really bad attack of flu and felt like death,' admits Mary. 'I couldn't fancy a cigarette all the time I was ill and by the time I felt better I hadn't smoked for three weeks . . . so I just never started again!'

So what would it take to make *you* give up smoking? Perhaps the first important question to ask yourself is why you smoke. What does smoking do for you, and can you find a safer, healthier way to get the same benefits? Perhaps you smoke because:

- you think it helps you to relax;
- you think it keeps you slim;
- it's something you do 'just for you' and you feel you deserve a little treat and a break from your work and domestic responsibilities;

- it's a habit – you automatically light up with a cuppa, or when you're enjoying a drink in the pub with friends.

A way to relax?

You may be surprised to read that smoking doesn't actually help you to relax. Look back to page 25 where I've described the effect smoking has on your heart rate and blood pressure. When you smoke those levels all go up, not down. What smoking does is calm the nicotine cravings. If you're really addicted there have probably been times when you have had to rush away from wherever you are – out of the office, out of the restaurant – and grab a cigarette. That's how stressful smoking can be.

You need to find other ways to help yourself to relax. Take a look at Chapter 9 of this book where we will be looking at stress and relaxation. There are other ways to calm your nerves. They include simple things like deep, even breathing or a cup of soothing herbal tea with a spoonful of honey. You can stroke your cat, listen to a favourite CD, go for a brisk walk or a swim, telephone your best friend or your partner, sing along to the car radio if you're driving, scream and punch a pillow in the privacy of your own home. The list is endless.

The truth about smoking and weight gain

One of the most common reasons why women – especially young women – take up smoking and go on smoking, is because they think it will help to keep them slim. It's true that smokers tend to be thinner than non-smokers and that when you give up smoking you may very well put on a little weight. However there are several factors you should take into account. One is that the amount of weight gained is likely to be very small, something like two or three kilos. Pay a bit more attention to what you eat and how much you exercise and you can soon lose that. Many ex-smokers, especially those who did not smoke a great deal, find that their weight stabilizes anyway as time goes by.

It is also true that the effect of smoking on the body's endocrine system means that smokers tend to store body fat around their waists and in their upper torso, rather than around their hips. Smokers, therefore, tend to have a higher waist-to-hip ratio or WHR than non-smokers. A high WHR is associated with a higher risk of developing heart disease, as well as other health problems. Pear shapes tend to be healthier than apple shapes! Swedish health researchers have looked at the distribution of body fat in smokers and ex-smokers and have found that putting on a little weight after giving up smoking is less of a health risk, because the weight is less likely to be deposited in the upper part of the body.

We don't yet know exactly *why* people put on weight when they give up smoking. It may be because smoking raises the body's metabolic rate and so burns calories more quickly, *or* acts as an appetite suppressant, so that people who have given up tend to eat more.

There is some evidence that giving up smoking using maximum-strength nicotine gum, nasal sprays or lozenges can reduce any associated weight gain.

You need to think carefully about the whole issue of weight. It's true that obesity is unhealthy, but the few pounds you may gain are unlikely to pose a health risk – and certainly not as much of a health risk as continuing to smoke! And if you think, as so many of us do, that staying slim equals looking good, ask yourself how attractive you look with a fag dangling from your lower lip, nicotine-stained fingers and teeth, bad breath, a smoker's cough and clothes that smell of stale cigarette smoke . . . need I go on?

If you think of cigarettes as your one 'treat', it might not be too difficult to think of something else that would give you just as much pleasure. Ask non-smoking friends what *they* do to wind down. Take a look at the relaxation tips in Chapter 9 and also remind yourself of how much you are spending on your smoking habit. Give up, and you could soon afford some pampering at a beauty salon, a meal out, a weekend break, or even a holiday, instead.

Smoking as a habit is becoming more and more difficult and anti-social with so many places banning it outright. Changing your everyday routine might help here, so you don't find yourself doing the same things or visiting the same places as you did when you smoked. Even having your cuppa in another room, with a magazine to concentrate on instead of a cigarette, might help you break the habit. If you need something to fiddle with while you answer the phone, play with a biro or get some worry beads. If you always buy your cigarettes in the same supermarket, shop in another. If you always call in at the same newsagents' on your way to work, vary your route – anything to help yourself to realize that things have changed now that you're a non-smoker.

What's the best way to give up?

This is the sixty-four-dollar question. The answer is that what suits one smoker might not suit another. Some swear by going 'cold turkey'; others use nicotine replacement patches or chewing gum; still others find hypnotherapy or acupuncture helpful. There are new drugs like Zyban and NHS 'Stop Smoking' clinics which offer the help and support, not just of health professionals, but of other people who are giving up at the same time. Whichever method you choose one thing is for sure:

> You won't be able to give up unless YOU really want to. You'll need a supportive family, partner and friends, and giving up will benefit them as well as you, but at the end of the day it has to be YOUR decision.

Finding the support you need

When you decide to give up, you could consult your GP for details of Stop Smoking clinics in your area, or alternatively call the NHS smoking helpline (contact details on page 98), or QUIT (contact number on page 99). According to the Royal College of Nursing, successful quitters are those who are motivated, understand their reasons for smoking, plan how they are going to give up, know what to expect when they stop, have support from friends and family, take it a day at a time, avoid situations where they are likely to lapse, and see themselves as non-smokers.

Olivia

Olivia was a 20-a-day smoker from the age of 16 until she was 22.

> I had a nasty attack of bronchitis and when I tried to smoke, my chest really hurt, so I decided to stop. I managed to cut down to one or two a day and then saw an ad for a Harley Street hypnosis clinic promising a 95-per-cent success rate. It cost £100. There were four of us in the room and we lay back while the therapist told us why we didn't want to smoke and asked us to imagine having healthy bodies instead.

Twenty minutes after I left I was dying for a cigarette again! But perhaps it had some effect because I didn't go back to 20 a day. Then six months later a friend of mine taught me some visualization exercises. I learned to relax properly and visualize the cravings being beaten by my wish to be clean and pure and full of energy. After a few weeks the addiction disappeared and I haven't smoked since.

Helpful products, therapies and drugs

No one can tell you how hard it will be for you personally. Everyone's experience is different. There are lots of products to help you give up if you don't trust yourself to 'just stop'. You can obtain advice on these from your GP or pharmacist. A *Health Which?* survey advised not believing exaggerated claims for these products such as 'quick, easy and painless' or '95-per-cent success rate!' Products include various forms of nicotine replacement therapy (NRT) in the form of patches, tablets or gum, non-nicotine gum, herbal and dummy cigarettes. Complementary therapies like acupuncture and hypnotherapy seem to work for some people, though there is little scientific evidence to support them. There is also the drug Zyban (buproprion hydrochloride), which is only available on prescription and is not suitable for everyone, but seems to help many smokers to give up.

'All our counsellors are trained to give advice which is tailored to the individual woman and her needs,' says a spokeswoman for QUIT.

Callers can ring their counsellor as often as they like. In fact, we find many pick up the telephone when they would otherwise have picked up a cigarette! The right way to give up can depend on a woman's age or her lifestyle. However we do know that drugs like Zyban, if it is appropriate for you, and various forms of nicotine replacement therapy, can double your chances of giving up successfully.

'I tell people who come to my clinics never to give up on giving up,' says Gay Sutherland, who runs the smoking cessation clinic at London's Maudsley Hospital.

Nicotine is a very, very addictive drug. Even teenagers who have only just started smoking may have withdrawal symptoms when they give up. If you're a 20-a-day smoker, you are taking 240 puffs a day, which means that 240 surges of nicotine are hitting your brain. For most smokers, nicotine is entwined in their lives. They automatically reach for a cigarette when they want to concentrate, when they pick up the phone, when they relax with a coffee or when they're in the pub with friends. It's an addiction – but like all addictions, it can be beaten.

The most successful ways to stop, for most women, are with a combination of medication like Zyban with behavioural support from a specially trained health professional. Smoking cessation clinics, which you can find out about from your GP or pharmacist, will typically offer once-a-week sessions for about seven weeks. You'll be asked to set a 'quit date' and then offered strategies to help you through the first four weeks. After that, the worst withdrawal symptoms will have subsided though you might still notice cravings, an increase in your appetite, and some weight gain.

Millions of women have successfully given up smoking, and so can you. There is evidence that successful quitters:

- are motivated by care for their health, concern about the cost of smoking, or increased social disapproval;
- are confident that they will succeed and have the support of non-smoking friends and family;
- feel that it's the right time for *them* to give up – perhaps a special birthday, New Year, or the start of a new relationship.

New drugs

More help is on the way for those who are determined to quit. At least two new drugs, varenicline and rimonabant, are currently undergoing trials, with promising results. Varenicline is a drug which mimics the effect of nicotine on the brain, and may make smoking less enjoyable. Rimonabant seems to work on different brain receptors and may also help smokers to give up. If the trials continue to go well both should be available in two or three years' time. Researchers are also working on a possible vaccine which will make smokers' bodies produce antibodies to nicotine, another way of making smoking less enjoyable. More effective NRT products with faster absorption rates are also in the pipeline.

5

Eating for a healthy heart

This chapter was going to be called 'Diet' but *diet* is such a miserable word. It conjures up a picture of deprivation, starvation, unhappiness, and above all something that is temporary. A 'diet' is something you try to put up with for a couple of weeks to fit into that lovely new bikini you bought for your summer holiday – and something you give up with a sigh of relief when you manage to squeeze into it.

Healthy eating, and especially *heart-healthy* eating, isn't like that. It's not about depriving yourself, it's about eating as much tasty, nutritious food as you need. It's not about starvation or self-denial. It's certainly not about unhappiness. Healthy people have a much better chance of being happy than people who always feel below par. And it certainly isn't temporary, because if you want to look after your heart, you need to get used to an eating plan that you can live with on a permanent basis. Not all at once, of course. It's asking too much to expect someone who has previously lived on a diet of fast food, cakes, sweets and loads of alcohol, to give it all up overnight for a regime of lettuce leaves and herbal tea. But you can get used to cutting down on the unhealthy snacks and increasing your intake of foods that are good for your heart.

There is clearly something very wrong with the way many of us eat in this country. Doctors are now talking about 'the obesity epidemic' and warning us that we are bringing up a generation of podgy, couch-potato children who are likely to die before their parents. It's a scary thought. Levels of obesity in both men and women have tripled since 1980 and there seems to be no sign of a slowdown in this upward trend. The Food Standards Agency claims that about half of British women are either overweight or obese. Obesity leads to 18 million sickness days off and about 30,000 deaths in Britain every year. Many of these deaths will be weight-related. It's a simple fact that if you are carrying loads of excess weight for your height and build, you are putting extra strain on your heart.

Take a look at the 'ideal weight' tables and you'll see that the recommended weight for a woman of, say 5 ft 4 in. should be no more than nine-and-a-half to ten stone (if you think in metres and kilograms, the equivalent figures are 1.63 m and 80 kg). If you weigh significantly more than that, it would certainly benefit your heart to lose a few kilos. Note, this doesn't mean you need to starve yourself to be supermodel-skinny. There is a big difference between a *healthy* weight and a *fashionable* weight, and most of us don't have the build of a Kate Moss or Jodie Kidd. If you are broad-shouldered and big-boned, you will naturally tend to weigh more than someone of the same height who has a more delicate frame. However you shouldn't make that an excuse to let the pounds creep on. Most of us know, deep down, when we need to lose weight.

You could also try working out your 'body mass index' (BMI), which is the figure you obtain by multiplying your weight in kilograms by your height in metres, squared. A healthy BMI is somewhere between 20 and 25, with 25-plus being overweight and over 30 being seriously overweight or obese.

However, experts now believe that for optimum heart health a more significant figure is your waist-to-hip ratio or WHR (see the chapter on smoking, pages 28–9). It seems that the traditional British pear-shape is a healthy one as far as your heart is concerned. People who put on weight around their middles, the apple-shapes, are more likely to suffer from coronary heart disease. This may be one reason why men, who tend to develop beer bellies, suffer from heart disease more than women, who tend to put on weight around their bottoms and thighs. If you have a waist measurement of more than 32 inches (80 cm), your health could already be at risk and if it is more than 35 inches or 88 cm, your risk of heart problems is much higher.

What is a heart-friendly eating plan?

Fortunately for us, a great deal is now known about heart-friendly foods. In order to take care of your heart you should be eating:

- less fat, especially saturated fats (see below);
- less salt – a maximum of 6g a day;
- more fruit and vegetables – a minimum of five portions a day and more if possible;
- more carbohydrates – things like bread and pasta – to stop you feeling hungry;

- smaller amounts of meat, cheese, nuts, and dairy products, low-fat where possible;
- far fewer puddings, cakes, sweets and sugary snacks. These should be occasional treats.

Within these guidelines it's very important that you eat a balanced diet, with foods from all food groups – proteins, carbohydrates, *some* fats, low-fat dairy products, fibre and antioxidant-rich fruit and veg, so that your body obtains all the vitamins, minerals and other nutrients it needs.

The good news is that a heart-friendly diet is also the kind recommended for a steady and sensible weight loss. 'Fad' diets, which involve cutting out whole food groups (such as carbohydrates) are not recommended, either for weight loss or heart health. For one thing, it's really boring to have to exist on such a limited range of foods, and for another, you are likely to miss out on vital nutrients. A small research study at Oxford University found that people on the once-fashionable 'Atkins diet' deprived their hearts of energy. The medical director of the British Heart Foundation was quoted as saying that extreme, unbalanced diets are a major insult to the body's metabolism and may have effects on the heart. In addition, the Atkins diet is very high in saturated fats.

Follow the guidelines above and you will lose weight slowly and steadily. You will also protect your heart. If you need more help, contact one of the slimming organizations like Weight Watchers (details on page 100) or Slimming World (address on page 99) for advice on healthy weight reduction and the support of like-minded slimmers.

A word about fats

The fat found in the foods we eat comes in four main types – saturated fats, poly- and mono-unsaturated fats, and trans fats – all of which have different effects on the body's cholesterol levels (see page 37 for more information about cholesterol).

Saturated fats

These are mostly found in animal-derived products like meat and dairy products, many of which – like lard and butter – are solid at room temperature. Some vegetable oils like palm oil and coconut oil are also high in saturated fat. Saturated fats raise the level of blood cholesterol, which has a negative effect on heart health.

Poly-unsaturated fats

These are found in some margarines (check the label!), plant oils, seeds and oily fish. They can lower the levels of LDL (bad) cholesterol but if you eat too much of them, they can also lower the level of HDL (good) cholesterol. They also reduce the levels of triglycerides (another form of fat) in the blood. Until recently it was thought that eating plenty of oily fish could reduce the risk of CHD since fish oils contain essential fatty acids like Omega-3 and Omega-6. However, an overview of the evidence recently published in the *British Medical Journal* showed no clear benefit. The BHF says that a varied and balanced diet is the sensible approach and that people should not stop eating oily fish or Omega-3 fats as there is no clear evidence either way.

Mono-unsaturated fats

These are found in some margarines (check the label), rapeseed oil, avocados, olive oil, peanuts and almonds. They lower LDL cholesterol without also lowering HDL.

Trans fats

Sometimes listed on food labels as trans-fatty acids or hydrogenated vegetable oils, trans fats are found in processed foods including margarine, cakes, biscuits, snacks and pastries. They are formed when vegetable oils go through a chemical process called hydrogenation, which was invented in the early twentieth century to give fats a longer shelf life. Evidence suggests that these fats raise LDL cholesterol and lower HDL cholesterol so they are best avoided.

Shopping and cooking wisely

It is easier than it has ever been to adapt your normal diet to make it lower in fat and more heart-friendly. All supermarkets now sell low-fat versions of everyday foods like milk, cheese and yogurt. Trim the fat off meat, and the skin off chicken. Bake or grill rather than frying your food. If you do choose to fry, use the smallest possible amount of olive oil rather than a 'hard' (saturated) fat like lard.

Always check the labels on margarines and spreads to make sure they are genuinely high in un-saturated fats. Specially produced spreads like Benecol do help to lower cholesterol, but so does a Mediterranean-style diet including plenty of oily fish and olive oil. If you really can't resist butter, make a point of spreading it really thinly and resist the temptation to add a knob of butter to your vegetables.

Vegetarians and heart health

You don't have to give up meat altogether to have a healthy heart, but there is some evidence that vegetarians are less likely to suffer from obesity and high blood pressure, both big risk factors for heart disease. It was thought that this may be because vegetarians tend to be slimmer. However, a new large-scale study led by Professor Paul Elliott of London's Imperial College suggests that there may be something in vegetable protein, possibly amino-acids or the mineral magnesium, which helps to lower blood pressure.

Scientific studies over the last twenty or thirty years seem to confirm that vegetarians have better heart health, on average, than meat-eaters. It has sometimes been suggested that this may be because vegetarians are generally more conscious of their health and fitness and lead healthier lifestyles. This is not necessarily the case. Researchers have found that even when healthy, fitness-conscious vegetarians are compared with equally healthy non-vegetarians their risk of CHD is smaller.

A vegetarian diet is generally a heart-friendly diet, unless you replace meat with a lot of high-fat products like cheese. Animal products are the main sources of dietary saturated fat, so avoiding these means that your overall fat consumption is likely to fall. A balanced veggie diet contains plenty of fruit, vegetables, wholegrain cereals and pulses, which are all recommended for optimum heart health.

The Vegetarian Society (contact details on page 100) sends out factsheets and booklets on healthy and heart-friendly eating.

Understanding cholesterol

Most of the cholesterol in the body is made in the liver and is used to make the body's cells, steroid hormones and Vitamin D. In addition, it helps to produce bile acids which help the body to digest and absorb fats. Cholesterol is also found in certain foods, for instance shellfish, offal, and egg yolks. Eating moderate amounts of these foods won't make much difference to your overall cholesterol levels, however. The body needs some cholesterol to fulfil these functions. What it does not need is too high a level of the wrong, or harmful, kind of cholesterol.

'Bad' cholesterol

About two-thirds of the cholesterol found in our bodies is the 'bad' kind – LDL cholesterol. We do need some of this, but having too much in the blood can lead to the fatty build-up which clogs up the arteries leading to atherosclerosis – the condition which leads to angina and heart attacks.

'Good' cholesterol

The other third is 'good' cholesterol – HDL cholesterol – which carries the 'bad' cholesterol away from the arteries and back to the liver.

Testing your cholesterol

A simple blood test which your GP or practice nurse can perform will tell you what your cholesterol levels are. Because these levels are affected by diet, you will be asked to fast for a few hours before the blood test. You will be given a result measured in mmol/litre. According to Heart UK, latest guidelines state that ideally your total cholesterol level should not be above 4 mmol/litre.

It is now thought that the important factor for heart health is the ratio of HDL or 'good' cholesterol to the total. If you ask your GP for a cholesterol test, make sure you ask for a full breakdown of your cholesterol levels. It can be useful to know the total level but what you really need to know is:

- the total which should be 4 or less;
- the HDL level which should be 1 or more;
- the LDL level which should be 2 or less;
- the triglyceride (see below) level which should be 2.3 or less;
- the ratio which should be 4 or below.

Bear in mind that these are ideal figures. You can have cholesterol levels slightly above this and still be perfectly healthy. If you have other risk factors for heart disease, such as a family history, or diabetes, then it's especially important to get your cholesterol levels as near to these ideal figures as you can.

Changing your diet can lower your levels of LDL and raise your levels of HDL cholesterol, meaning that your arteries are less likely to clog up. High cholesterol causes no symptoms so you need the blood test before you can decide whether your diet needs adjusting. If it does, as well as the commercial 'cholesterol-lowering' products you see on the supermarket shelves, you can help yourself by eating more garlic, fruit and vegetables, wholegrains, soya and oats.

Heart UK point out that products like Benecol and Flora Pro-Activ can only help as part of a generally heart-friendly lifestyle. In other words, using them will not protect you from heart disease if you continue to eat unhealthily and take no exercise. Supplements such as garlic perles are also available. They can be useful if you really don't like garlic but it's perfectly possible for most people to lower their cholesterol levels simply by changing the way they eat.

LDL cholesterol levels can also be affected by stress, according to a new study by researchers at University College, London. For more information on ways in which stress affects your heart, see Chapter 9.

If changing your diet doesn't lower your cholesterol levels sufficiently, or if you are at high risk of heart problems (i.e. you are diabetic or have already had a heart attack) your doctor can prescribe cholesterol-lowering medication too. (See Chapter 10.)

About triglycerides

If you have had your blood cholesterol levels checked, your triglyceride levels should have been checked as part of the same test. Triglycerides are another type of fat, which are found in foods like meat and dairy products. The fat stored in the tissues of the human body is also made up of triglycerides. As with cholesterol, it's important to have low levels of these fats in your blood, no more than 2.3 mmol per litre. Higher levels are associated with an increased risk of heart disease.

Levels of triglycerides rise after a meal, especially a fatty meal.

Recommendations for keeping the levels healthily low are similar to those for cholesterol, for example:

- maintaining a healthy body weight;
- drinking alcohol only in moderation;
- cutting down on fats, especially saturated fats, and spreading your consumption of fats throughout the day;
- cutting down on the amount of sugar you eat;
- eating several servings of oily fish per week. Omega-3 fatty acids, found in fish oil, have a beneficial effect on triglycerides.

About homocysteine

As long ago as the 1960s, a Harvard Medical School pathologist studied children who suffered from severe heart problems at a young age and discovered that they had very high levels of a toxic protein called homocysteine in their blood. It seems that people who eat a lot of animal protein tend to have high levels of homocysteine, as do people with CHD. The amount of homocysteine an individual produces is influenced by her diet and also her genes, and can be measured by a simple blood test. Men are, however, more at risk, as are smokers and people with kidney damage. You can ensure that you have healthy homocysteine levels by eating plenty of folic acid, a vitamin contained in vegetables like broccoli, spinach, sprouts and other dark green, leafy vegetables, citrus fruit, pulses, wholegrains and fortified breakfast cereals. Folic acid supplements are also available.

Alcohol and your heart

The good news is that you can continue to enjoy a drink and still have a healthy heart. The bad news is that Britain's binge-drinking culture, where young women, in particular, drink in order to get as drunk as they can, as often as they can, is the worst possible scenario for heart health.

Alcohol affects heart health in several different ways. Most alcoholic drinks are high in calories and low in nutrients, so if you drink heavily you will find it difficult to lose weight. A pint of lager has 160–180 calories, a gin and tonic 130, a glass of red wine between 80 and 100. Sweet drinks like alcopops, some liqueurs and many mixers have a high sugar content, which again adds calories to your total intake.

The current healthy drinking guidelines advise that women should drink no more than two or three alcohol units a day. A 'unit' of alcohol would be a small glass of table wine, half a pint of ordinary-strength lager, or a single pub measure of spirits. It's also recommended that you have at least two, and preferably three, alcohol-free days every week. Don't save up your weekly allowance of 14 units to 'spend' them all on one almighty binge at the weekend which, alas, is what some women tend to do.

How does alcohol affect the heart? The most obvious way is by raising blood pressure. Drinking alcohol is the second most common cause of high blood pressure, after obesity, and high blood pressure is a major risk factor for heart disease. According to the charity Alcohol Concern, binge-drinking is especially associated with raised blood pressure. They define binge drinking, for women, as drinking more than seven units of alcohol in one session. If it seems unfair that men, with their generally heavier bodies and higher total body water, can get away with drinking more, well, that's just the way it is!

There is some good news. It seems that moderate alcohol consumption, within the 14-units-or-less-per-week safe limits, is actually good for the heart. It's thought that this may help to explain the so-called 'French paradox'. French people traditionally eat lots of high-fat dishes – think of all those buttery croissants and tasty liver pâtés – but they also drink more sensibly than we do, use lots of olive oil in cooking, and eat plenty of fresh vegetables. Women (and men) who drink about one unit a day are at lower risk of heart disease. However this doesn't seem to apply to *every* woman, only to those who are at risk of heart disease anyway – which means older women who have already gone through the menopause. Younger women's hearts are not likely to benefit from drinking at this moderate level, and young women who drink *more* than one or two units of alcohol a day are putting their health and well-being at risk in all kinds of ways.

6

Exercise and your heart

Apart from eating a healthy diet, the other half of the 'heart-health' equation is exercise. Doctors are already concerned about the growing rates of obesity and inactivity among Britons. Not only are we eating too many fatty and sugary foods but we are also not working off the calories with sensible amounts of exercise. Too many of us, it seems, don't do any exercise *at all*. This applies particularly to women. Surveys suggest that almost four out of ten women don't even have *one* 30-minute period of activity per week, when at least 30 minutes per day is recommended – and more, for those who can manage it. As far as risks to heart health are concerned, lack of exercise comes way up at the top of the list. About a quarter of British women smoke, about a third have high blood pressure, but as many as *three-quarters* don't get enough exercise to protect their hearts. As a result, it has been estimated that as many as six out of ten women can't maintain a 3 mph walking speed up a 5 per cent slope.

Think about it. In our grandparents' day, far more people walked or cycled to work, or at least walked to the bus stop or train station. Now, too many of us have a car parked in the drive and a car park outside the office or factory. Women shopped in small local shops every day and trudged home carrying their shopping baskets. No once-a-week trips by car to a massive out-of-town supermarket for them! Housework used to be a whole lot more labour-intensive. Think of all that hand washing, mangling, pegging sheets and towels out on a washing line instead of popping them into the tumble dryer. Rugs were dragged out into the backyard and beaten. Doorsteps and floors were scrubbed, not wiped over quickly with a squeegee. Work was physically harder, too – more stairs and fewer lifts, more manual typewriters and no computers. Physical activity was far more of a part of women's daily lives than it is today.

Why does that matter? Well, the heart is a muscle, and like all muscles it becomes weaker if it isn't efficiently used. Basically, the more you work your heart muscle, the stronger it becomes. More blood is pushed round with every heartbeat and more oxygen is delivered to your muscles, enabling them to contract more easily.

The fitter you are, the slower your 'resting heart rate' or RHR. Your RHR is measured in 'beats per minute' (bpm) and a fit person's RHR will be something like 50–60 bpm. An averagely fit person has an RHR of around 72 bpm and and an unfit person's RHR is somewhere around 80–90 bpm. In order to become fitter and lower your RHR, you need to take part in aerobic or 'cardio' exercise. This is the kind which uses large muscle groups like the legs, is rhythmic and repetitive, burns calories, warms you up and makes you breathe more quickly as well as raising your heart rate. Good examples of aerobic exercise are:

- brisk walking
- jogging
- fast swimming
- rowing
- dancing
- cycling
- exercise or step classes
- using exercise machines like treadmills or stationary bikes at the gym.

You can check your own resting heart rate by counting the beats of your pulse for ten seconds and then multiplying the figure by 6 to calculate the average number of beats per minute. A heart-rate monitor is a more efficient way of measuring how fit or unfit you are, and will give you an idea of how best to work your heart efficiently. One of the advantages to joining a gym or working with a personal trainer is that it will help you to work out just how much cardiovascular exercise you should be doing, and at what intensity, to give your heart a safe and effective workout. Generally, you should be working out at a rate that is between 65 and 85 per cent of your 'maximum heart rate' or MHR. For women, the maximum heart rate is held to be 226 minus your age in years. So, if you're 40, your maximum heart rate is 186 bpm. If you haven't exercised before, though, you should start at a lower level, something like 50–55 per cent of your MHR, increasing as you become fitter.

How exercise affects your heart

As well as helping your heart to pump more efficiently, exercise helps your cardiovascular system in other ways. Fit women are less likely to develop high blood pressure than unfit ones. If you do have high blood pressure, a sensible exercise programme can help you to lower it.

We all know that, in combination with a sensible eating plan, exercise can help you lose weight. And, just as women who are fit are less likely to develop high blood pressure, they are also less likely to develop diabetes. Women with diabetes are about four times as likely to get CHD than women without it. Regular exercise also seems to raise the level of HDL or 'good' cholesterol in the blood. Physical activity can also help to prevent blood from clotting.

Everyday fitness

You don't have to join an expensive gym to get fit. Although, of course, if you fancy the idea, go along to your local gym and see if they do 'induction days' which will show you what a gym workout is all about, and whether or not it's for you.

Says Clare Wheeler, Divisional Manager at Fitness First, which has 166 clubs around the UK including 13 'Fitness First for Women' clubs:

> Women often have the misconception that health and fitness clubs are full of Lycra-clad, muscle-bound men and women who are all extremely fit and know exactly what they are doing. However, at Fitness First we welcome a wide range of ages, shapes and sizes.
>
> The aim of a fitness professional like me is to welcome everyone into the club and to help, support and guide members to achieve their goals. We understand that people feel nervous in a new environment, therefore ensure that qualified professionals are on the gym floor to help members relax and enjoy their time with us.
>
> A health club provides a warm, friendly, safe and relaxed environment to work out in and achieve the personal results you are looking for. The fitness professionals are on hand to help members make a difference to their lives, and that is the reason why we all joined the fitness industry!

However, if you really believe the gym is not for you, there are many ways you can incorporate more exercise into your everyday life.

> The most important thing about any exercise regime is that you should enjoy it!

That really is Rule One – in fact, it's one of the most important rules. If you take up any form of exercise you don't enjoy, it will become a chore and you won't keep it up. So find something you like doing. There must be something!

Remember, your initial goal should be 30 minutes a day of moderately strenuous exercise. That means exercise that is strenuous enough to leave you feeling a little warm and breathless, but not so breathless that you can't carry on a normal conversation.

If you have any doubts about your health, check with your GP first and let her know that you are thinking of taking up an exercise regime. The chances are she will tell you to go for it and that it can only benefit your heart and your whole cardiovascular system. She might also remind you that exercise has other benefits, like lowering your blood pressure, raising the level of good cholesterol in your blood and lowering the level of bad cholesterol, reducing your risk of developing diabetes, helping you to maintain a healthy weight, preventing osteoporosis by strengthening your bones, relieving stress and helping to reduce both anxiety and depression.

There are lots of ways you can incorporate more exercise into your everyday life before you even start thinking about joining a gym, taking up a sport, buying a fitness video or joining an exercise class. You can start with something that's cheap, easy, and that anyone can do – which is walking.

Walking – the perfect exercise?

We can't all be ace tennis players or graceful dancers, but we can all walk. Even if you think you are too busy for an exercise regime (and who are you kidding?), you can include some walking in your day no matter what your circumstances. If you normally drive (or are driven) to the station in the morning, then walk instead. If you normally drive the kids to school, you would all benefit from the walk. If you normally take a bus, then walk to a bus stop further from your home and get off a couple of stops from the office. If you're based at home, walk to the shops, the kids' playgroup, the childminder. Don't buy your daily paper at the corner shop, walk to the High Street and get it instead.

Take yourself out for a walk at lunchtime and eat your sandwiches in the park. If you're meeting friends for the evening, walk to their place or the pub or the cinema. Walk into town for shopping, or take a bus there and walk back – this halves your fares too! And at the weekends take yourself and the family out for a walk instead of spending your free time slumped in front of the TV. Walk the dog. If you don't have a dog of your own, busy neighbours will probably be delighted if you offer to walk theirs, as might any local Animal Rescue organization. Some Councils actually organize guided walks for people who want to increase their fitness but don't much fancy walking alone. Contact the Council's sport or recreation department and see if there's anything in your area.

Explore your local area. See if the library has books of local walks. You will be surprised how many places of interest there are when you start to investigate the town you live in. Or, take a bus or the car to a local beauty spot or country park and walk from there. It doesn't matter where you go, it doesn't even much matter what the weather's like. Wrap up warmly if it's cold, wear weatherproofs if it's wet, carry water-bottles if it's hot, make sure you all have comfortable shoes – just get walking.

If you haven't exercised before, the BHF recommends that you start by walking for just 10 or 15 minutes at your normal walking pace, two or three times a week. Do this for a couple of weeks. In the next fortnight, go out for the same length of time but quicken your pace on your return journey. Increase both your speed and the number of walks you take in the fifth and sixth weeks, and go for slightly longer, brisker walks in the seventh and eighth weeks. By Week 9 you should be able to walk briskly for 30 minutes, five times a week – your basic fitness target. More, of course, is even better!

Finding exercise to suit you

What about other forms of exercise? Some women were put off sport at school by being forced to take part in team games or activities they didn't enjoy. There are so many forms of exercise you can choose from, though, there is certainly something you would enjoy; it's just a question of finding it.

You'll need to ask yourself a few basic questions. Do you like the idea of being in a team or playing with other people, or are you happier exercising on your own? Do you like the outdoor life, or are you better indoors? What about music, would that encourage you to work out? Are there games and sporting activities you've longed to try but never got round to, or thought they weren't appropriate for someone your age, or your size? The local Council's Leisure Department is sure to be able to offer you all kinds of choices, just call them up. They often run exercise classes aimed at older or less fit women, and sometimes classes exclusively for women. Sport England is an organization dedicated to getting couch potatoes up and moving (contact details on page 99).

Here are some ideas to get you started. Have you thought about taking up:

jogging, keep-fit, aerobics, step classes, trampolining, fencing, basketball, badminton, tennis, swimming, aqua-aerobics, women's football or rugby, ballroom dancing, line-dancing, salsa, country- or folk-dancing, golf, cycling, rambling, spinning, Pilates, power-walking, dry ski-ing, Nordic walking, Boxercise, ballet, Fitball, rowing, netball, disco or jazz dance, ice-skating, kick boxing, martial arts, rollerblading, snowboarding, hockey, Body Conditioning, skipping, squash, hiking, pole-dancing, British Military Fitness, Slimnastics, lacrosse, table tennis, climbing, scuba-diving?

There is almost bound to be something on that list which appeals to you! And that's without mentioning the possibility of buying a fitness video which enables you to work out in your own front room, or a piece of exercise equipment that turns your garage or spare room into a home gym.

Start slowly

If you haven't exercised before, or for a long time, then *do start slowly*. Do five or ten minutes of bending, stretching, and 'stepping' on the spot before you begin your workout proper. This increases blood flow to your muscles and helps to avoid damage to ligaments, muscles and tendons. Don't risk sprains and strains. It's equally important to 'cool down' after your workout with a few moments of gentle, steady marching on the spot until your heart rate returns to its resting level. A few simple stretches help, too. Exercise is not supposed to hurt. If it does, stop. Don't push yourself beyond your limits, especially not at first. Muscles you haven't used for some time may feel a little stiff the day after you begin an exercise programme, but you shouldn't be in agony, or unable to move.

If you already have heart disease ...

You may be surprised to discover that exercise can still help you! People who are physically active are at only half the risk of developing CHD, compared to the inactive. If you have a heart attack, the fact that you have been physically active makes it more likely that you will survive. Rehabilitation programmes for heart attack patients all include physical exercise as it reduces your risk of dying, or of having another heart attack. (See Chapter 11 for more information about rehabilitation after a heart attack.)

You should talk to your GP, cardiac nurse, or hospital doctor about the type and amount of exercise you can safely do if you have heart disease. You will normally be told that exercise will help you, except in the case of particular heart conditions such as hypertrophic cardiomyopathy (see page 10), aortic stenosis (a narrowing of the heart valves) or if exercising brings on palpitations, causes severe chest pain or breathlessness, or leads to dizziness, fainting or nausea.

Most people with common heart conditions such as angina will be encouraged to exercise. It's especially important to *start slowly* and build up gradually to the level of exercise recommended by your doctor. Angina, as we have seen, occurs when the heart is unable to deliver enough oxygen, causing chest pain. Steady, regular physical activity will improve the blood supply to the heart muscle, meaning that the heart has to work less hard and less pain is experienced.

If you have angina and you find that exercising brings on the pain you will find it helpful to use your GTN spray or tablet (see Chapter 10) before exercising. The BHF recommends putting a tablet under your tongue or using one dose of the spray and letting it dissolve. The pain should go within five minutes; if it doesn't, you can take a second dose, and even a third. After three doses, if the pain does not go, you should dial 999.

The BHF also advises those with angina to avoid the kind of competitive sport which requires bursts of intense activity, heavy manual work outside when it's cold, and exercising after a heavy meal. All these forms of activity put an extra strain on your heart. Be guided by your doctor's advice; she knows your particular circumstances. Building up gently to a regime of 30 minutes of moderate-intensity activity each day is a good way to maintain and improve your cardiac fitness.

Walking is an excellent form of exercise for anyone with angina, heart failure, or high blood pressure because you can start with just a few minutes' gently paced walking and work up gradually until you are walking further and faster. If walking brings on chest pains, makes you breathless, or leaves you feeling exhausted, you may be trying to do too much, too soon. Don't overdo it. Once you are comfortably walking for 20 or 30 minutes a day, you could consider taking up another activity, such as swimming, dancing or perhaps cycling.

Sex and your heart

Might a night – or several nights – of passion be as good for your heart as a 5 km run or a workout at the gym? Sadly, there's no real evidence that people with good sex lives are at lower risk of heart attacks, though like any form of exercise that increases your heart rate, making love is good for you!

If you have a heart condition or you have had a heart attack, you and your partner might be worried about resuming your normal sex life afterwards. Sex does increase the heart rate and raise the blood pressure, giving the heart more work to do, and may lead to worrying symptoms like chest pain and breathlessness. The BHF says that sex is usually considered to be safe if the person can:

- walk about 300 yards on the level without getting chest pain or becoming breathless
  OR
- climb two flights of stairs briskly without getting chest pain or becoming breathless.

As with any form of exertion, sex can bring on angina in some people and the same advice applies – keep your GTN spray or tablets by the bed and use them if this is the case with you. Some of the drugs routinely given to cardiac patients may affect your sex drive. If this is a problem for you don't be too shy to ask your GP or cardiologist about it. There's no reason why you should have to give up a normal, loving sex life just because you have a heart condition.

7

Hormones

One piece of good news for heart health is that being a woman means that you are at lower risk of coronary heart disease than a man, all other factors being equal. This is because female hormones have a protective effect on the heart, at least up to the time of the menopause when oestrogen production slows down. According to British Heart Foundation figures, only 34 women under 35 died of CHD in 2003, compared with 135 men in the same age group. In the 45–54 age group, the figures are 685 for women and 3,198 for men. It's not until women reach the 75-plus age group (when they far outnumber men in the general population) that the number of deaths from CHD is greater in women than in men (40,990 as against 34,744).

The Pill and heart health

Ever since hormonal contraception, such as the Pill, was introduced in the 1960s there have been many studies looking at the long-term effects. These have included looking at women's risk of developing blood clots and high blood pressure while on the Pill and mean that your GP or family planning clinic will need to know your medical history – and the history of your family – before prescribing the Pill for you. Serious side effects are rare, but you need to be sure that this form of contraception is suitable for you.

The 'combined' Pill contains two hormones, oestrogen and progestogen, which are similar to the natural hormones women produce. A very few women who take it may develop a blood clot which can block a vein or artery. Women at increased risk of this happening include those who:

- are smokers, especially if they are over 35;
- are diabetic;
- are very overweight;
- have high blood pressure;
- have a close blood relative who suffered a thrombosis or heart attack before they were 45;
- already have heart disease.

However, contraceptive choices are a highly individual matter and there's no one-size-fits-all answer. If you have any of the risk factors mentioned above, hormonal contraception will not necessarily be ruled out for you. It could be that a lifestyle change, for instance giving up smoking or losing excess weight, will enable you to take the Pill as normal, and it's something you should discuss with your doctor.

A spokesman for the Family Planning Association advises:

As a general rule, we say the cut-off point for using the combined Pill is 35 if you are a smoker, but healthy non-smokers can continue to use the Pill up to the time of the menopause. The Pill's suitability is to do with each woman's general health history and lifestyle rather than her age.

The progestogen-only Pill, sometimes known as the mini-Pill, is another very efficient form of contraception. It works in a slightly different way from the combined Pill and doesn't contain any oestrogen. However, it may not be recommended for you if you have an existing heart condition or very high blood fat levels.

Other hormonal methods of contraception such as the injection (Depo-Provera or Noristerat) or implants (Norplant) contain the hormone progestogen, like the mini-Pill. Again, they may not be suitable for you if you have heart problems, but you should discuss their suitability with your doctor.

If you are using any form of hormonal contraception it's important that you have regular check-ups from your GP or clinic so that your weight can be monitored, your blood pressure checked, and any problems you may be having with side effects can be discussed.

Pregnancy and heart health

Pregnancy is, of course, a perfectly natural process, but it does put extra strain on the heart. The average woman will put on between 22 and 28 lbs or 10 to 12.5 kg during pregnancy, though it varies a lot from woman to woman. In the last three months of pregnancy, a woman's heart rate can increase by as much as 10 to 20 beats per minute as the heart works harder to cope. The volume of blood in a woman's body increases by as much as 40 to 50 per cent during pregnancy and her heart has to work harder to pump all this extra blood around. Routine ante-natal check-ups sometimes reveal an extra heart sound because of this. For most women, it causes no problems, though a few may be referred to cardiologists if they are thought to be at risk of complications. This all underlines the fact that if you are planning a pregnancy, you owe it to yourself and your baby to become as fit and healthy as you can be – giving up smoking, making exercise part of your everyday routine, and eating the healthiest possible diet. A healthy lifestyle won't just protect your own heart, it will give your baby the best possible protection against developing coronary heart disease in later life.

Women with congenital heart disease

Advances in the care of babies born with heart conditions – which may affect one in a hundred babies – mean that a whole generation has survived problems which would have killed them forty or fifty years ago. Many heart defects in babies are picked up by routine ultrasound scans during the mother's pregnancy. Others are not discovered until the baby is born, or even later in life. There may be holes in different parts of the heart, blood vessels may be narrow or wrongly placed, or the valves between the chambers of the heart may be faulty. Most of these conditions can now be corrected surgically and allow people to lead normal or near-normal lives.

However, if a woman has grown up with congenital heart problems she will need special care during her own pregnancy. A few women with particular conditions may be advised to avoid pregnancy altogether.

According to current thinking from the BHF, women who know they have heart problems should be referred to an obstetrician, ideally before they become pregnant. Every woman's circumstances will be slightly different but anyone who has had heart surgery will be under close observation during her pregnancy. Pregnant women with congenital heart disease will want to discuss the possibility of the baby inheriting the same condition. Mums-to-be taking blood-thinning drugs like warfarin run an increased risk of excessive bleeding during labour and birth, so need to be especially carefully monitored.

The GUCH (Grown Up Congenital Heart Patients Association – contact details on page 97) can offer help to women with congenital heart problems, both from health specialists and other women in the same position. They offer a useful leaflet on pregnancy and point out that:

- pregnancy in women who have congenital heart problems should be carefully planned. You may have to adjust the medication you are taking for your heart condition before becoming pregnant;
- you should see both a cardiologist and an obstetrician to discuss your care during pregnancy and exactly what the risks are to your own health;
- like all women planning a pregnancy you should take care of your health;
- if you have a congenital heart condition, there is a chance your baby may also have one. The risk is roughly 1 in 20; for women without heart problems the risk is 1 in 111. Your baby will be scanned in the womb as soon as possible so that any problems can be identified at an early stage;
- depending on your own health, your baby is slightly more at risk of being 'small for dates' or of being born prematurely;
- it's especially important that you receive regular check-ups from both your obstetrician and your cardiologist as your pregnancy progresses;
- labour and birth are usually safe for women with heart conditions though you are slightly more likely to have a forceps, suction cup or Caesarian delivery and may be advised to stay in hospital slightly longer than usual. You will be given antibiotics to prevent endocarditis when labour begins.

Hormone Replacement Therapy (HRT) and heart health

The average age of menopause – specifically, the date of the last period – in the UK is 51, but some women have their final period in their mid-forties and others not until their mid-fifties. Others have an early menopause, either naturally or because of surgery to remove the womb and/or ovaries (hysterectomy). At that time, the ovaries stop producing female hormones.

Symptoms of the menopause

As well as the obvious effect of periods stopping, women may suffer from a variety of symptoms including:

- hot flushes and night sweats;
- vaginal dryness which can make sex uncomfortable;
- loss of interest in sex;
- mood swings;
- lack of confidence;
- anxiety and panic attacks.

Few women are unlucky enough to be affected by *all* these symptoms. Even individually, though, they can be upsetting enough for women to seek help from the medical profession. In addition to the menopausal symptoms that women notice, changing hormone levels are having an effect on women's metabolism at this time and this can, in its turn, affect heart health. For instance, menopausal women tend to:

- have higher levels of LDL or 'bad' cholesterol;
- have higher levels of triglycerides in their blood;
- be less able to process glucose and insulin;
- put on weight round their middles, i.e. become 'apple-' rather than 'pear-shaped';
- have rather thicker blood which clots more easily.

All these factors increase the risk of heart problems in later life, and seem to be linked to the loss of female hormones which happens at the menopause.

Long-term effects of HRT

Replacing natural hormones with synthetic ones in the form of 'Hormone Replacement Therapy' should, in theory, protect older, post-menopausal women against heart disease, and HRT was recommended to many women in order to do just that. However, recent large studies of the long-term effects of HRT on women's health seem to suggest that the answer is not quite that simple.

The hormone oestrogen was first identified in the 1920s and a synthetic version was being produced by the 1930s. Forty years ago, when HRT was first introduced for menopausal women in the USA, it was seen as a miracle treatment for older women. Not only did it stop the hot flushes, it was also recommended to prevent osteoporosis, benefit heart health, and keep women young and lively! Some doctors and their older female patients still feel that way about it. HRT can undoubtedly help some women to cope with the uncomfortable and sometimes distressing symptoms of the menopause. It was also originally thought to have a protective effect against heart disease by replacing the body's natural hormones. At least 30 research studies suggested that HRT benefited women's heart health. The oestrogen it contains does appear to increase the levels of HDL or 'good' cholesterol and lower the levels of LDL or 'bad' cholesterol.

However, more recent and extensive studies in both Britain and the USA have suggested that this may not be the case. A major report in 1998 found that women on HRT actually had higher rates of heart attacks than those on placebo pills in the earliest years of the trial. In later years the risk seemed to drop, so overall there was no difference. Another report in 2000 which had studied women with pre-existing coronary heart disease found that HRT didn't improve their overall heart health, even though it did seem to lower LDL cholesterol. An even bigger study of 26,000 women without a previous history of CHD found that heart attacks, strokes and blood clots were more common in women taking HRT in the early stages of the research.

Weighing up the risks and benefits of HRT

The jury still seems to be 'out' on the precise benefits HRT can offer to individual women. Some doctors feel that the large American studies referred to above looked at older, less healthy women who had taken high doses of HRT for many years and that the findings were not necessarily relevant to prescribing patterns in the UK. However, current thinking from the Royal College of Obstetricians and Gynaecologists is that HRT *does not* protect against heart disease. They say that if it is prescribed it should be at the lowest possible effective dose to improve menopausal symptoms, for the shortest possible time.

HRT can certainly help women who suffer from severe menopausal symptoms. It can also help to prevent the bone-thinning disease osteoporosis. As HRT does not seem to protect against heart disease in the long term, it should not, therefore, be prescribed for cardiovascular protection in women who don't have menopausal symptoms. A conference of the International Menopause Society in 2000 also recommended that women who already have heart disease probably should not take HRT.

The Society felt that for most women at the time of menopause, lifestyle changes such as giving up smoking, taking more exercise, eating a heart-friendly diet and, if necessary, taking cholesterol-lowering drugs (see Chapter 10) were better ways of improving heart health than taking HRT.

It seems that as far as most women are concerned, as with many drugs, it is up to each individual and her doctor to work out the risks and benefits of taking HRT in her particular case.

The BHF is supporting research into how declining hormone levels may affect women's hearts and circulation. Their Head of Medical Information said in December 2005:

Hormone replacement is helpful for some women who are finding it difficult to manage the symptoms associated with the menopause. There is no clear evidence in humans that hormone replacement and the contraceptive pill decrease the risk of heart disease, and therefore they should not be prescribed to protect women's hearts.

We should be clear that fatty build-up can develop in the arteries from puberty in both men and women. Therefore it's vital that young people reduce their overall risk of heart disease from an early age, by eating a healthy diet, controlling their weight, physical activity and not smoking.

Diet and the menopause

Women who are unable to, or don't want to take HRT, can often be helped through the menopause by dietary changes such as those recommended by the Women's Nutrition Clinic (see contact details for Natural Health Advisory Service on page 98). As clinic founder Maryon Stewart says, women of menopausal age can now expect to live for another twenty-five or thirty years, so need to find an effective way of maintaining healthy hearts during that time!

In addition to the standard advice offered to older women about giving up smoking, watching their weight, eating a heart-friendly diet and exercising, the Women's Nutrition Clinic has other suggestions for improving their heart health. In her book on 'natural' menopause treatments (details on page 100), Maryon Stewart points out that both menopausal symptoms and increased heart disease seem to be characteristic of Western communities and are much less common in China and Japan. Chinese and Japanese diets are traditionally lower in meat and dairy products and higher in pulses, vegetables, oily fish and above all, soya products.

Soya

Researchers as long ago as the 1960s discovered that soya seemed to lower cholesterol levels. A later analysis of 40 published studies on the subject found that 34 of them had showed that soya in the diet produced at least a 15-per-cent drop in LDL or 'bad' cholesterol levels. Subsequent studies found that soya could also increase HDL or 'good' cholesterol. It is now known that soya, as well as some seeds like flax, sunflower, pumpkin and sesame seeds, plus pulses like chickpeas and lentils, contain phyto (or plant) oestrogen, a substance which is similar in effect to the natural oestrogen produced in women's bodies, but less powerful. Phyto-oestrogens have a similar effect and can balance the body's own levels of hormones after the menopause, leading to an improvement in menopausal symptoms. In both the USA and Britain, it is now accepted that food products containing soya may, in conjunction with a low-fat, low-cholesterol diet, protect against heart disease. Supplements containing soya isoflavones (a type of phyto-oestrogen) are widely available in chemists and health food stores and soya products like milk, yogurt, desserts and spreads can be found in all major supermarkets. Japanese people, who have the highest life expectancy in the world, consume about 50 to 100 mg of isoflavones per day, compared with the average Western consumption of 30 mg or less.

8

Diabetes

Diabetes – or 'diabetes mellitus', to give it its full name – is a relatively common condition in which the pancreas, a gland which lies just behind the stomach, is unable to produce the insulin the body needs to control the amount of glucose in the blood. In what is known as Type 1 or 'insulin-dependent' diabetes, there is a severe lack of insulin which has to be replaced by injection. This type of diabetes usually develops in people under the age of 40, sometimes in childhood, but more often at puberty. The second, more common type of diabetes, Type 2 or 'non-insulin-dependent' diabetes, usually develops in older people. In this type, either the pancreas is still producing some insulin but not enough, or the body is unable to process the insulin properly. The end result is the same – too much glucose in the blood, which the body is unable to convert into energy in the normal way. Type 2 diabetes is usually treated with drugs and a change of diet, though insulin injections sometimes have to be given.

Exactly what causes diabetes is not yet known. There is certainly a genetic element involved, as people with a family history of diabetes are most at risk of developing it. Research is still going on into why some members of families develop diabetes and others don't. Overweight people, and those of African-Caribbean and South Asian origin are also at higher risk. According to Diabetes UK, about 80 per cent of those people diagnosed with Type 2 diabetes are overweight, but that still leaves 20 per cent who are of normal weight. Increasing levels of obesity in the population mean that more and more of us are being diagnosed as diabetic. In fatter people, insulin is simply unable to do its job. A few women develop diabetes during pregnancy, so-called 'gestational diabetes', and women who suffer from polycystic ovary syndrome are also at higher risk.

There are special implications for heart health, as it's known that both men and women with diabetes are at higher risk of CHD. This is because the high levels of glucose in the blood of diabetics make the blood stickier. Either the cells clump together in the form of blood clots and travel round the system, or they stick to the walls of the arteries, making the arteries narrower. This, in its turn, means

59

that the heart has to work harder to pump the blood through the narrowed arteries, and blood pressure increases. About 3 per cent of the population has diabetes, but between 10 and 15 per cent of those admitted to hospitals with heart attacks have the condition. About 20 per cent of those who die from heart attacks are diabetics. According to British Heart Foundation figures, women with Type 2 diabetes have a three- to five-fold annual risk of CHD compared with non-diabetics. Diabetes UK estimates that women with diabetes are eight times more likely to die of cardiovascular disease (heart attack or stroke) than women without diabetes.

This can sound frightening, but although diabetes can't be cured at present, it can be treated and controlled. Leading a healthy lifestyle by giving up smoking, eating a heart-friendly diet, and doing plenty of exercise, can reduce the risk for diabetic women as well as those who do not have diabetes. Perhaps because of the increasing number of very overweight people in our population, the incidence of diabetes is increasing. Statistics from the British Heart Foundation show that the prevalence of diagnosed diabetes in women has increased by a massive 80 per cent since 1991. There are probably around 2.5 million people with diabetes in the UK today. Many of those have not been diagnosed and so are unable to take the steps that would allow them to take better care of their health. All diabetes is serious and needs to be taken seriously and treated properly, for the sake of your heart health as well as your general fitness.

Symptoms of diabetes

So how would you know if you had diabetes?

The symptoms include:

- needing to pass urine much more often than usual, especially at night;
- increased thirst;
- excessive tiredness;
- losing weight when not dieting;
- some women suffer from recurrent thrush;
- visual disturbances like blurred vision.

If you suffer from any of these symptoms, and especially if you know there is diabetes in your family, ask your GP to test your blood sugar levels. This can be done by a simple blood test. Diabetes is *not* caused by eating too many sweets, it is not infectious or contagious, and it's not caused by stress, although stress can worsen the symptoms in some people.

Making lifestyle changes

Having diabetes not only puts you at higher risk of heart problems in itself, but also magnifies the effect of other risk factors, such as smoking, being overweight, having higher than normal cholesterol levels and high blood pressure. If you have diabetes, you owe it to yourself to make appropriate lifestyle changes, not only to help manage your diabetes, but also to protect your heart.

Basically, a healthy diet and lifestyle for a woman with diabetes is very much the same as a healthy diet and lifestyle for a woman who doesn't have the condition. It's even more important that you give up smoking if you're a diabetic, and you should also pay careful attention to your diet and take plenty of exercise.

The charity Diabetes UK, which campaigns on behalf of diabetics and funds research into the condition, has a helpline offering advice on lifestyle changes for those with diabetes (contact details on page 96). Advice nurse Cathy Moulton has these suggestions for women with diabetes who are concerned about heart health:

There's no blanket advice on diet which is appropriate for everyone with diabetes. A lot depends whether the patient has Type 1 or Type 2 diabetes and whether or not she is being treated with insulin. Generally though, the advice on healthy eating is the same as for non-diabetics. Meals should be based on complex carbohydrates with reduced amounts of salt, sugars and fats. Five portions of fruit and vegetables a day are recommended. A woman who is on an insulin regime might need to adjust what she eats. Life for diabetics is no longer ruled by meal times, as it used to be. Insulin pumps are available to deliver a measured dose at all times. A woman on oral medication also needs to eat healthily and if she is planning to lose weight she should watch how much carbohydrate she takes in.

A woman newly diagnosed with diabetes should liaise with health professionals to work out an eating regime which is appropriate for her as an individual. Many GP surgeries now have practice nurses specially trained in the management of diabetes.

As far as exercise is concerned, nothing is ruled out! If your diabetes has led to any complications, for example if you have very high blood pressure, you should discuss any exercise regime with a health professional. Here at Diabetes UK we have had members climbing Kilimanjaro and running the London Marathon! Diabetic athletes need to plan their training regimes very carefully. For example anyone running a marathon needs to work out when they will need a snack or a sugary drink as it is very important for diabetics to keep their blood sugar controlled. Exercise will use up the body's store of glucose so that athletes may be at risk of a 'hypo' for as long as 15 hours after exercising. [Hypoglycaemia or 'hypo' is the medical term for a low blood glucose level, which can lead to symptoms like trembling, sweating or palpitations. It is treated by taking some short-acting carbohydrate such as a sugary drink or snack.] Diabetic athletes may need to plan a bit more carefully than other people if they are taking part in the more extreme forms of exercise, but ordinary exercise such as walking, swimming or cycling is fine.

Medication for diabetes

As well as insulin, diabetics are often treated with drugs whose job is to help the body process glucose efficiently. Sulphonylurea drugs like glibenclamide or gliclazide stimulate the cells in the pancreas to produce more insulin. Other anti-diabetes drugs work in a slightly different way. Metformin changes the way in which the body metabolizes sugar. Acarbose slows the digestion of starches and sugars and so helps to regulate blood sugar levels after a meal. According to Diabetes UK, there are no particular problem interactions between these drugs and those prescribed for heart conditions. Indeed, some of the drugs which are prescribed to treat high blood pressure, notably the ACE inhibitors and angiotensin II blockers, are recommended for diabetics as they protect against possible kidney damage. (See page 79 for more information about these drugs.)

It's worth remembering that not all drugs suit every patient. If you are prescribed one for diabetes or high blood pressure which causes unacceptable side effects, it may be possible to alter the dose or change to another drug which will suit you better.

Hormone replacement therapy and diabetes

As insulin is itself a hormone, diabetics can be sensitive to hormone treatment. Depending on her medical history, it may be possible for a women with diabetes to benefit from HRT, if she is suffering from severe menopausal symptoms. There are several different kinds of hormone treatment, some oestrogen-only, some including progestogen, and different ways of delivering the correct dose including tablets, patches and pessaries. Deciding whether to take HRT has to be an individual choice made between a woman and her medical advisers. It is also worth considering natural therapies for menopausal problems. For more information about appropriate diets and supplements, contact the Women's Nutrition Clinic (see contact details for Natural Health Advisory Service on page 98).

Leah
Leah, 56, has had diabetes since she was a child.

As a child I couldn't just run out and play with the other children because I got tired quickly and my legs ached. I also wasn't allowed sweets, so I felt I was missing out.

I didn't know about the connection between diabetes and heart disease and when I began suffering from chest pain, I really didn't associate it with heart problems. Then one day when I was on holiday I collapsed with chest pain and was rushed to hospital, where it was found that I had had a heart attack. I was put on medication at first, which didn't seem to help. Eventually I was transferred to Guy's Hospital in London where I was given an angioplasty. Unfortunately the pain came back after three months and I had to have another. Now I've had a total of three operations, the most recent a year ago, and I've been doing really well since then.

I have now learned to look after myself. I exercise a lot, between one and a half and two hours every day. I go to the gym and have an exercise bike at home which I use while I am watching TV. I also eat a very healthy diet with no hard fats or fried food, and have lost two and a half stone in weight. A balanced diet with regular meals is very important for diabetics. I can even eat a few sweets now, and I've been able to reduce my dose of insulin to a child's dose.

These days I don't feel good if I don't exercise. I only wish I had taken it up before!

9

Stress and high blood pressure

Stress is a fashionable buzz-word these days. We're no longer describing ourselves as worried or anxious, we're 'stressed-out'. Not that stress isn't a very real problem for many of us. It has been estimated that stress-related health problems lead to the loss of 12.8 million working days per year in Britain and cost the economy a whopping £4 billion. We live in a fast-moving, fast-changing world and that has an impact on stress levels, especially for women. Many of us end up doing an endless juggling act. We are coping with a job or career, a relationship, a family, perhaps the demands of elderly relatives, money worries, the pressures of a consumer society which hints that we haven't made it if we're not cooking superb meals, going on wonderful holidays, wearing fabulous clothes and treating our kids to the latest gadgets. No wonder some of us occasionally feel that it's time to slow down ...

Not that stress is necessarily a bad thing. Some stress, in the form of excitement, interest and motivation, is what it takes to get us up in the morning. One woman's stress factor is another woman's welcome challenge. Some women are able to cope with what are apparently high levels of stress, like Nicola Horlick, the top businesswoman who has also had six children. Hearing about women who manage to 'have it all' can make the rest of us feel inadequate and guilty if we sometimes find it difficult to cope with our own less high-powered lives, and that can be stressful in itself.

The British Heart Foundation acknowledges that stress can play a part in the development of heart disease even though the exact mechanism by which this happens isn't always known. The BHF recognizes four particular causes of stress:

- Work stress – which, perhaps surprisingly, can affect women more than men. We tend to think of stress as affecting top executives with excessive responsibilities, but according to BHF research the most stressful thing about work is 'not feeling in control'; which affects the lower-paid and less powerful employees. An extensive, 14-year study of 10,000 civil servants by researchers at University College London, published in the *British*

Medical Journal in January 2006, found that people who reported the most work stress were more likely to develop both heart disease and diabetes. The most stressed-out had high cholesterol, high blood pressure and 'apple-shaped' figures, which, as we have seen, do pre-dispose to heart problems. Women were five times more likely to develop these risk factors than men were.

- Lack of social support – in other words friends, family and people to confide in. Here women tend to do better than men.
- Depression and anxiety, both of which affect both men and women.
- Particular personalities, notably those who seem to have a lot of anger and hostility in their psychological make-up. 'Type A personalities' – the kind who are ultra-competitive, often high achievers, do everything very quickly, are impatient and easily angered – are about three times as likely to have heart attacks as more laid-back characters!

Stress affects different people in different ways. Obviously-stressful events like bereavement, redundancy or the break-up of a relationship can cause all kinds of physical, mental and emotional symptoms: anything from insomnia, headaches, mysterious aches and pains, digestive disorders, to anxiety attacks and depression. One study of 199 healthy middle-aged people carried out by University College London found that stress led to a rise in the levels of LDL or 'bad' cholesterol which could persist for as long as three years. Even welcome and happy events like a house move, a new job or the birth of a baby can prove to be stressful. Some people turn to damaging behaviours like smoking or excessive drinking as a way of coping. Later in this chapter we shall be looking at healthier and more effective ways of reducing stress.

What stress does to your body

We are all primitive cave-dwellers at heart! When faced with a threat from a sabre-toothed tiger or woolly mammoth, the reaction of primitive man or woman was to engage in what is known as the 'fight or flight' syndrome. At moments of extreme stress and anxiety, hormones, including adrenaline, pour into the bloodstream. The heart rate increases, blood pressure rises, more blood flows to the muscles and more air enters the lungs to prepare the body for a life-or-death physical struggle or a dash to safety. It's all about survival and in extreme circumstances it's exactly what is needed. However, most of the stress factors in our lives today are not a matter of life and death. We don't really need those surges of hormones or those sudden increases in heart rate and blood pressure, and they can, in fact, be damaging. High blood pressure is one of the most important risk factors for heart disease.

More about blood pressure

Stress isn't the only cause of high blood pressure, but it can contribute to it. Blood pressure is the measure of the force which is exerted on the walls of your arteries as your blood is pumped around your body. When you have your blood pressure measured, you are given two figures. The systolic pressure is the reading when your heart beats, and the diastolic pressure is when the heart relaxes in-between heartbeats. Blood pressure is measured in millimetres of mercury, and written down as 'mm Hg'. The blood pressure of a normal, healthy adult should be less than 140/90 mm Hg – often expressed as 140 over 90.

About a third of women in Britain have blood pressure which is higher than normal, many without knowing it. As well as stress, causes of high blood pressure include being overweight, drinking too much alcohol and smoking. Eating an unhealthy diet and not getting enough exercise can also contribute. High blood pressure can run in some families and members of the African-Caribbean community are especially at risk. The British Heart Foundation says that every 20 mm Hg increase in systolic and every 10 mm Hg increase in diastolic pressure actually doubles the risk of CHD (and other health problems as well, including stroke illness). It's recommended that people with diabetes should try to keep their blood pressure below 135/85.

Age is also a major risk factor for high blood pressure. Only about 2 per cent of young people between 16 and 24 have it, compared with about two-thirds of the over-65s. Whatever your age, you should have your blood pressure checked regularly just to make sure that all is well.

High blood pressure doesn't usually cause any symptoms, or not until it has reached a level dangerous enough to cause chest pain or breathlessness. Lifestyle changes are often enough to lower blood pressure. Your GP will recommend:

- keeping your weight at a healthy level. A recent study of more than four and a half thousand people in four countries found that a diet rich in vegetables, pulses and grains tends to produce lower blood pressure;
- reducing the amount of salt you eat – don't add salt at the table or in cooking and cut down on salty snacks like crisps and salted nuts;
- giving up smoking, which narrows the arteries and makes the heart work harder;
- sticking to the recommended guidelines on healthy drinking – not more than one or two units of alcohol a day and no binge-drinking;
- learning to relax more (see below for more tips on relaxation).

If this sort of lifestyle change is not enough to lower your blood pressure, you may be prescribed medication, which is extremely effective. For more information on blood pressure medication, see Chapter 10.

Low blood pressure

Don't worry if, when you have your blood pressure taken, the figures are low, with a systolic reading of around 100. According to the Blood Pressure Association, low blood pressure is a healthy sign for almost everyone and reduces the risk of a heart attack in later life. However, if you experience symptoms like faintness or dizziness when changing position – getting up from a chair, for example – you should mention it to your GP. The chances are that it's unimportant, but for a tiny minority of people it could be a sign of some underlying problem that needs investigation.

Are you getting enough sleep?

It is very much easier to cope with the stresses and strains of daily life if you are getting a good night's sleep – but are you? Most people suffer from insomnia at some time, and up to a third of us claim to be chronic poor sleepers. Much insomnia is caused by stress and anxiety – and ironically, the less well you sleep the more anxious and stressed you are likely to be! Lack of sleep has a general stress effect on the body with rising levels of the stress hormone cortisol in the bloodstream.

There's no 'right amount' of sleep for everyone. Sleep experts say that if you wake up refreshed and ready for the day ahead, you are getting enough sleep whether you've been in bed for four hours or nine. Sleeping pills can only ever be a short-term answer to insomnia. Many of the relaxation therapies mentioned in this chapter should help if you have trouble sleeping.

Simple ways to reduce the stress in your life

There are as many ways of winding down from everyday stress as there are women! For some, even the daily commute can be a stress-buster, rather than a stress-inducer, as 51-year-old Laura explains.

Laura
I have a half-hour drive to the office every day. Instead of using the dual carriageway I make a point of travelling along country roads. I have a CD player in my car and I put on some favourite music and just sing along. My mobile is switched off and I think of that half-hour as 'me' time, when neither my husband, my two teenagers or my colleagues at work can reach me. Modern communications mean we are now expected to be in touch at all times but I think that's a recipe for stress. If they can't manage without me for half an hour, morning and evening, it's just too bad!

Laura's attitude is a healthy one. So many women simply try to do too much – both at work and at home – instead of learning a few basic time-management skills that would enable them to cope better with the demands of the day. If you feel stressed because life seems to be getting on top of you and there never seem to be quite enough hours in the day, try sitting down and making a list of all the things you have to do:

- today
- this week
- in the next six months.

Today's list could include doing the laundry, going to work, shopping for tonight's dinner in your lunch hour, meeting a friend after work, taking your daughter to Brownies, cooking dinner, writing a report for work, walking the dog, writing and posting a birthday card for your Mum, washing your hair.

This week's list could include the rest of the housework, a major shop, ironing, booking a dental appointment, taking the car for its MOT, buying and posting a birthday card to your Mum, introducing a new member of staff at work to her schedule, going out to dinner with friends.

The 'six-months' list could include applying for promotion, choosing and booking your holiday, getting something done about the leaking roof, tidying the garden, planning the new kitchen you've been dreaming of, arranging a surprise party for your partner's birthday . . . and so on and so on.

Now, look at those lists again. Are you surprised you're feeling stressed? Borrow the kids' coloured crayons and put red stars by all the tasks you absolutely have to do, and blue crosses by the ones someone else could do perfectly well. That will leave you with some which – whisper it – *don't have to be done at all*. Stop trying to be a superwoman. There's no such thing, and you will run yourself ragged even attempting it. Women were not born with a steam-iron in one hand and a duster in the other. All household tasks can be shared, and no one wants to live on a film-set anyway. It's amazing how quickly men and boys learn how to iron a shirt when they realize that if they don't, their shirts remain un-ironed! Similarly, many work tasks can be better organized, or delegated to someone else.

Stress-busters

There are plenty of books on household management and quick cooking for busy women. Once you have off-loaded some of the unnecessary demands on your time, how are you going to use it to de-stress properly? Quick, easy everyday stress-busters can include:

- a long, hot bath, perhaps by candle-light, with your favourite bath oil.
- a blockbusting novel and a glass of wine.
- laughter. It has been proved that laughter can banish stress, so watch a comedy video.
- pets in your life. We can all learn a lot about relaxation by watching a sleeping cat. Dentists sometimes have tanks of tropical fish in their waiting-rooms to calm nervous patients' fears.
- music – either a favourite CD or a specially devised relaxation tape.

- plants and flowers. Scientific studies have shown that hospital patients recover more quickly when they can see trees from their ward window, and blood pressure drops when people walk in woodlands.
- gentle exercise produces endorphins, the body's own feel-good hormones.
- a massage by your partner, maybe leading to a comforting cuddle or even a love-making session. Touch is amazingly therapeutic, as is good sex.
- an absorbing hobby. Men seem to be better at what is sometimes known as 'the potting-shed syndrome' when they switch off from everyday worries by retiring to the potting shed. Golf and gardening play the same de-stressing role. Isn't there something you could become just as absorbed in – a craft like pottery, an amateur dramatic group or choir, a collection that gets you rooting about for bargains in junk shops and car-boot sales?
- a sense of perspective. Many of the everyday things that wind us up and raise our blood pressure are not really *that* important. When you feel your stress levels rising, ask yourself how much it really matters that you're stuck at a red traffic-light or you've had to wait ages in a bank or supermarket queue? That's the time to take a few deep, relaxing breaths, let those tense shoulders drop, and take yourself to . . .
- a 'happy place'. There must be somewhere – a favourite holiday beach, your own comfortable bed, an armchair by the fire – where you feel completely relaxed. When things get too much for you, close your eyes and imagine you're there. Feel the sand between your toes or the warmth of the blankets, listen to the waves or the crackling of the flames. Imagine your toddler's toothy grin, your partner's arms round you, your cat purring on your lap, and feel the tension drain away.

More ways of tackling stress

You might feel that you would benefit from a bit more direction in learning how to relax. Whether you normally use complementary medicines or not, you could consider some sort of complementary therapy to help you deal with stress. One of the main differences between complementary and conventional medicine is that complementary medicine works holistically; that is, it treats the whole person, not just the particular illness or injury. People are not machines. Many doctors now feel that this kind of 'integrated' medicine is the way forward. Complementary therapies like yoga, meditation, autogenic training, massage, hypnotherapy and others can decrease stress and aid relaxation.

Yoga

Yoga, for example, has been developed over thousands of years to promote good physical health and inner peace. The word yoga comes from a Sanskrit word meaning 'union' and yoga is designed to promote union between mind and body by the use of correct breathing, physical exercises and meditation. You don't have to be a contortionist and the best way to learn is to join a class.

Herbal medicine

At one time, all medicines were herbal medicines, and many of the drugs we use today, such as aspirin, were originally derived from plants and herbs. Health food shops stock herbal medicines from established companies like Potter's, whose range is the largest in Europe and includes Newrelax tablets for stress and tension and Nodoff to aid restful sleep. For a detailed diagnosis and personally tailored prescription, you will need to consult a qualified medical herbalist.

Bach flower remedies

Dr Edward Bach was a homoeopath who devised 38 special 'flower remedies' to be used for particular personalities and particular emotional states. Bach Rescue Remedy, widely available from health food stores and specialist pharmacies, is a composite of five flower remedies and is specially recommended for everyday stress and emotional crises.

Homoeopathy

This treats patients on the principle that 'like cures like' and uses individually prescribed remedies to treat the whole person, not just the symptoms. Homoeopathic remedies are widely available from pharmacies and you'll need to choose the one which best suits your personality and circumstances as well as your symptoms. For more detailed help, consult a qualified homoeopathic doctor.

Meditation

Different kinds of meditation – transcendental meditation or Buddhist meditation among them – can help those who practise it achieve a state of deep relaxation. Once you have been taught to meditate, twenty minutes twice a day can benefit conditions such as irritable bowel syndrome (IBS) and asthma as well as anxiety and high blood pressure. EEGs (electroencephalograms) have shown that meditation produces alpha-waves in the brain, associated with rest and relaxation.

Autogenic training (AT)

Devised by a German doctor in the 1920s, AT is similar to meditation and self-hypnosis. Patients are asked to repeat a series of simple instructions designed to promote deep relaxation and switch off the 'fight or flight' response. Introduced to Britain in the 1970s, AT has been scientifically proved to help stress-related conditions including high blood pressure.

Massage

This is probably the earliest form of therapy known to man. There are many different kinds with 'Swedish' massage being the best known. A massage therapist uses various different touching techniques to soothe out the 'knots' in tense muscles. Stroking, pummelling, tapping, knuckling and wringing may also be used, with or without the addition of calming essential oils.

Hypnotherapy

Hypnotherapy involves the therapist putting the patient into a trance-like state in which she is much more suggestible (though she can't be made to do things she wouldn't normally do!). There's plenty of evidence that hypnotherapy helps some people give up addictions like smoking, and it can also be useful in dealing with anxiety states and phobias, as well as stress-related conditions like IBS.

T'ai chi

This is a combination of gentle martial art, exercise and meditation. Like most Chinese therapies, it's aimed at balancing the body's 'chi' or vital force and promoting harmony and calm. 'Meditation in motion' is one description of this ancient art, which is now very

73

popular in Britain and is sometimes recommended as therapy for those who have had heart surgery, as well as anyone suffering from stress-related health problems.

Finding a therapist

It's important to find a reputable therapist with whom you feel comfortable. Make sure anyone you consult belongs to the appropriate professional organization such as the National Institute of Medical Herbalists (contact details on page 98). You'll find details of the governing bodies for many complementary therapies between pages 95 and 100. Personal recommendation is also a good way to find someone. You will normally have to pay, but more and more medical practices are referring patients to complementary therapists so you could ask your GP.

Coping with panic attacks

It is very easy to confuse the symptoms of panic with those of a heart attack. Panic attacks often come out of the blue and are a sign of extreme stress. Symptoms include a racing heart, breathlessness, chest pains, dizziness, numbness and tingling in hands and feet, and above all, a feeling of complete terror. If you have never experienced anything like it before it is easy to convince yourself there must be something seriously wrong and that you are going to faint, make a fool of yourself in some way, or have a heart attack and die.

The fact is that however distressing panic attacks are, *they are not dangerous.* Learning to cope with panic attacks means accepting that *nothing will happen to you.* Once you have learned to accept that – and it isn't easy, it's something you do have to learn, and you may need help to do so – you will find that the panics happen less frequently. It makes sense to go to your GP, explain what has happened and ask for a general check-up to make sure there is no physical reason for your symptoms. Once you have been given a clean bill of health, contact one of the self-help groups for phobics and panic-attack sufferers such as No Panic (contact details on page 98). They have helped thousands to learn to control their anxieties and they can do the same for you.

10

Living with heart disease

Earlier chapters of this book have mostly been concerned with
prevention – things that you can do to protect yourself and stop heart
disease developing. Whatever your age and family history, it always
helps to give up smoking, eat a healthy diet, and take plenty of
exercise. Sadly, for some people, prevention just isn't enough and
they find they have to learn to live with heart disease. It's true that
treatments are improving all the time. New drugs to treat heart
conditions are being developed and more is known about the most
effective way of taking the drugs we have. Some 200,000
prescriptions for drugs for heart conditions were dispensed in 2004,
more than four times the number twenty years ago.

Diagnosis and tests

Before any treatment programme is worked out, though, a proper
diagnosis needs to be reached. You and your doctors need to know
for certain what your problem is. Perhaps you have high blood
pressure, putting you at risk of CHD. This can be measured quickly
and efficiently by your GP or practice nurse at the doctor's surgery.
Depending on how high the reading – or readings in the plural,
because your doctor will want to check that you really do have
permanently raised blood pressure and are not just anxious about the
test itself – you may be offered diet and lifestyle advice or you may
be prescribed one of the range of blood-pressure lowering drugs,
which we shall be listing later in this chapter.

Or perhaps you have gone to your GP complaining of chest pains
or symptoms like breathlessness which makes her suspect that you
could be suffering from heart disease. In that case you will be
referred to your local hospital for tests, usually beginning with an
ECG (electrocardiogram). Some GPs are able to offer this test in
their surgery, but it's more common to have it in hospital.

ECG tests

An ECG is designed to discover whether there are any problems or
irregularities with your heart rhythm. It's a quick and simple test

which can also show if you have had a heart attack, whether this happened recently or some time ago. It's painless and involves having sticky patches called 'electrodes' attached to your chest, arms and legs. These are then wired up to a machine which registers the electrical signals coming from your heart and prints them on to paper.

An exercise ECG is just what it sounds like – the same test, but taking place while you are exercising on a running machine or perhaps an exercise bicycle. If you have been having chest pains when you exercise, this can show how activity affects your heart and exactly what the problem is. You will be asked to start running or cycling gently and the rate will then increase. If you get chest pains or become uncomfortable, tell the doctor or technician what is happening.

Twenty-four-hour ECG recording is recommended when you have irregular symptoms like palpitations. Again you are wired up to electrodes, but they are attached to a small recorder about the size of a personal stereo which you wear for 24 hours so that any changes or irregularities in your heart rate over that period can be noted.

Chest X-rays

A chest X-ray may be required if you have symptoms like breathlessness which can be caused by heart disease but by other conditions as well. You'll have to stand with your chest against a photographic plate which takes an X-ray picture of your heart, lungs and chest wall, so that your doctor can see if your breathing difficulties are caused by heart problems.

The echocardiogram

This works a bit like radar in submarines and bats! A probe is placed on your chest and a pulse of high-frequency sound is passed through the skin. It doesn't hurt at all. The probe picks up echoes from the various parts of your heart and shows them on a screen. An echocardiogram can show just how well all the parts of your heart are working, including the valves, and the way your heart pumps blood round your body. Sometimes echocardiogram pictures of the heart are taken from the gullet (oesophagus) by a tiny probe which you need to swallow. A 'stress echocardiogram' may be taken after the heart has been put under stress with exercise or drugs. Another possible test, called IVUS or 'intravascular ultrasound', is where a small probe is inserted into an artery so that the state of the artery walls can clearly be seen on the screen.

Radionuclide tests

Some hospitals use these tests to obtain more detailed information about how well the heart is working. They are less common than ECGs and echocardiograms. A small amount of a radioactive substance called an 'isotope' is injected into the blood and a camera picks up the gamma rays sent out by the isotope, creating a 'picture' of the heart's activity. Depending on the isotope used, the test may be referred to as a radioisotope scan, MPS, SPECT, technetium scan, thallium scan, MIBI or MUGA scan.

The PET scan

A small amount of radioactive material is again injected into your blood. You then have to lie for some time under a scanning device, so that doctors can see your blood flow and how your heart muscles are working.

Electrophysiological testing

A few specialist hospitals are able to offer this kind of test, which helps with the diagnosis of unusual heart rhythms and locates the part of the heart which is affected. Electrodes are inserted gently into the heart to record its electrical activity. An ECG can then often show whether medication is effective in treating the abnormal rhythms or whether a pacemaker needs to be fitted.

The MRI scan

This is another diagnostic tool only available in specialist units. The patient has to lie in a kind of tunnel around which there is a magnet. Magnetic fields and radio waves produce detailed pictures of internal organs including the heart. It can help to show how the heart and blood vessels are working and where there are abnormalities.

Cardiac enzyme tests

These are basically blood tests taken several times over the course of a few days to determine whether a patient has had a heart attack. After a heart attack, the levels of certain enzymes in the blood rise and can be measured. A similar test measures the levels of another protein called a 'troponin' to confirm whether or not there has been a heart attack.

The coronary angiogram

The tests above can give a great deal of information about the way your heart is working and what the problems might be. An angiogram gives a more detailed picture of where any narrowing of the arteries is, how well your heart valves are working and exactly how efficiently your heart is pumping blood around your body. A catheter – a long, narrow, flexible tube – is passed through an artery in your groin (usually, less commonly an artery in your arm), through your blood vessels and into your heart. At this time an ECG records your heart rate, heart rhythm and blood pressure. The procedure takes between 20 minutes and an hour. Your doctors will explain exactly what is happening, what you can expect, and what the risks are. An angiogram will help them to work out the most appropriate treatment for your particular heart condition.

Medication for heart problems

Because heart disease is so common, dozens of different drugs have been developed to treat it. Many people with heart conditions have a variety of problems – for example, high blood pressure, breathlessness, atherosclerosis, irregular heart rhythms, valve problems – so that they need to be prescribed several different drugs. The fact that there are so many drugs to choose from has its advantages. If you experience side effects, the chances are that your doctor will be able to change your medication to something else which doesn't cause you the same difficulties.

If you are prescribed medication that doesn't suit you, tell your GP or cardiologist. Don't just stop taking it or your symptoms may recur.

Drugs for high blood pressure

As we have already seen in Chapter 9, high blood pressure is a major risk factor for heart disease. It makes sense to keep your blood pressure under control, especially as most people with high blood pressure don't get any symptoms or warning signs that they have a problem.

Sometimes, simple lifestyle changes like losing weight, exercising more, drinking less alcohol or eating a healthier diet can have an effect on blood pressure. If these changes are not enough, medication will be prescribed. This can include:

- ACE inhibitors (examples: captopril, ramipril). ACE is short for 'angiotensin converting enzyme' – angiotensin being a chemical which narrows the blood vessels. ACE inhibitors relax and widen the arteries.
- beta-blockers (examples: atenolol, metoprolol). These drugs help to reduce blood pressure and slow the heart rate down by blocking the action of adrenaline, the 'fight-or-flight' hormone.
- calcium-channel blockers (examples: verapamil, nifedipine). Calcium is needed to help the heart muscle to work properly. A reduced amount of calcium allows the arteries to relax and widen.
- centrally acting hypertensives (example: methyldopa) act on the mechanism in the brain which controls the width of blood vessels.
- diuretics, including thiazides and loop diuretics (example: bumetanide) turn excess body fluid into urine, which is passed out of the body. This leaves the heart with a smaller volume of blood to pump around.
- alpha blockers (example: doxazosin) block the nerve signals which make blood vessels constrict.
- angiotensin II antagonists (examples: losartan, valsartan) work rather like ACE inhibitors (see above) in relaxing and widening the arteries.

Side effects of these drugs can sometimes seem troublesome, especially if your high blood pressure wasn't causing you any obvious problems before it was diagnosed. They can include dizziness and fainting, particularly at the start of treatment, as your blood pressure may fall excessively before the dosage is adjusted to suit you. Headaches, drowsiness, digestive upsets and a dry cough are also possible side effects. Adjusting the dosage, becoming accustomed to the drug, or changing to another one are all possible solutions.

The ASCOT study

According to the Blood Pressure Association (contact details on page 95), it may be more effective to treat high blood pressure with a combination of different drugs. A large international research study, the Anglo Scandinavian Cardiac Outcome Trial (ASCOT), looked at a total of 19,000 people in the UK and Scandinavia over a period of six years to find out what combination of medication was the most effective in preventing heart attacks in people with high blood pressure. The conclusion was that those who took an ACE inhibitor plus a calcium-channel blocker (see above for information on these types of drugs) *and* a cholesterol-lowering drug called a statin (see below for more information about statins) could reduce their risk of having a heart attack by more than half. This combination seemed to work equally well, regardless of the patients' cholesterol levels.

This doesn't mean that women who are currently being treated with other drugs for their high blood pressure should necessarily change. For one thing, the people in the study were treated with only *one* of each of the many calcium-channel blockers, ACE inhibitors and statins available. It's not yet known if the other drugs in the same 'families' would be equally effective. The study also found that those treated with a combination of a beta-blocker and a diuretic were slightly more likely to develop diabetes, another heart-disease risk. In future, beta-blockers may not be recommended as a 'first-choice' treatment for high blood pressure. However, they are also used in the treatment of angina and heart failure with great success.

If you have any questions about your medication, side effects or general effectiveness, continue to take it but ask your GP or practice nurse for more information on your next visit.

Cholesterol-lowering medication

As with high blood pressure, a change of diet can often help to lower cholesterol and so reduce your risk of heart disease. Again, not everyone can be helped by lifestyle changes so medication may need to be prescribed as well. A class of drugs called 'statins' are most commonly used to lower cholesterol. Another group of drugs called 'fibrates' can be used when statins are not suitable. Fibrates also lower the levels of triglycerides in the blood. A group of drugs called 'resins' are another possible treatment.

- Statins (examples: simvastatin, pravastatin) work by blocking a liver enzyme essential to the production of cholesterol in the liver.

The liver then takes the cholesterol it needs out of the bloodstream instead, lowering the level of LDL or 'bad' cholesterol in the blood by as much as 30 or 40 per cent and total cholesterol levels by 20 per cent.

In March 2006 an American study found that taking a very high dose of the most powerful statin could reverse the effect of furred-up arteries by shrinking fatty deposits. The BHF said that these results were encouraging but that more research was needed to discover whether this treatment would lead to fewer heart attacks.

- Fibrates (examples: bezafibrate, fenofibrate) are prescribed for patients with a combination of high cholesterol and raised triglyceride levels. They reduce the very low density lipoproteins in the blood and can lower triglyceride levels by up to 50 per cent and cholesterol by up to 25 per cent, while increasing levels of HDL or 'good' cholesterol by 10 or 15 per cent.
- Resins (example: cholestyramine) otherwise known as bile acid binding resins, work on the bile acids made in the liver, causing them to be passed out of the body. In order to make more, the liver has to draw more cholesterol from the bloodstream and the result is lower LDL cholesterol levels. Resins come in powder form and have to be mixed with liquid to be taken.

These drugs are generally well tolerated with minimal side effects, apart from some gastro-intestinal problems like nausea, constipation or diarrhoea.

Medication for angina

Drugs prescribed to treat angina include beta-blockers (see page 79) and calcium-channel blockers (see page 79) which, as we have already seen, may also be used to lower blood pressure. Other anti-angina drugs are listed.

- Nitrates (examples: glyceryl trinitrate, isosorbide dinitrate) dilate the blood vessels by relaxing the muscles in the blood vessel walls. These drugs come in the form of tablets which are dissolved under the tongue, patches and sprays to reduce the pain of angina. They also have a preventative effect.
- Potassium channel activators (example: nicorandil) are drugs first

introduced in the 90s which widen both arteries and veins to help with blood flow.

- Anti-platelet drugs (example: aspirin, clopidogrel) are used to help prevent clots forming in the blood. These drugs reduce the stickiness of the small blood cells called 'platelets' which can stick together to form clots. Aspirin is often prescribed for people at risk of, or already diagnosed with, coronary heart disease, but is not suitable for asthmatics or those with stomach ulcers.

Medication after a heart attack

Heart attacks (see Chapter 2) are caused by a blood clot blocking a coronary artery. Treatment for a heart attack will include drugs which relieve pain, as well as 'clot-busting' or thrombolytic drugs such as streptokinase. Aspirin is also given. Depending on the individual case, other drugs may be given later to prevent further heart attacks or to treat any complications.

Medication for heart failure

Several different drugs or combinations of drugs may be prescribed to deal with the symptoms of heart failure, such as breathlessness and fatigue. Diuretics (see page 79) may be combined with ACE inhibitors (see page 79) and also with digoxin, a drug originally derived from the leaves of the foxglove plant. Digoxin helps the heart to pump more efficiently, increasing blood flow to the kidneys and enabling excess fluid to be passed out of the body. Angiotensin II inhibitors and beta-blockers (see page 79) may also be used to treat heart failure.

Medication for arrhythmia

Minor disturbances of the heart rhythm, or palpitations, are common and often don't need any treatment. If medication is required one of the many heart drugs may be prescribed, including beta-blockers (see page 79), digoxin (see above) and calcium-channel blockers such as verapamil (see page 79). Other anti-arrhythmia drugs include:

- Amiodarone, which is very effective but may produce side effects such as headache, dizziness and stomach upsets. Regular blood tests are also required to check its effect on your lungs, thyroid and liver. This drug also makes the skin extremely sensitive to sunlight so you need to use plenty of sunscreen when taking it.
- Flecainide may be prescribed for serious disturbances of the heart rhythm.
- Propafenone is another anti-arrhythmia drug which is not, however, suitable for asthmatics or those with lung disease.

Medication for valvular heart disease

If you have a problem with your heart valves you may be prescribed ACE inhibitors (see page 79), diuretics (see page 79) or digoxin (see page 82). If you have valve replacement surgery you will need to take anti-coagulant drugs such as heparin or warfarin. These drugs are given to prevent the formation of blood clots either in the short or long term. Heparin is given by injection in hospital, often after surgery. Warfarin is taken in tablet form and while you are taking it you will have regular blood tests. Anti-coagulants interact with many other drugs, including aspirin and oral contraceptives, so tell anyone treating you for another condition that you are taking them.

Like all drugs, those prescribed for heart conditions can cause side effects, some more serious and/or uncomfortable than others. Because there are so many drugs available, you and your doctors may have to experiment with dosages and different types of drug before you find a regime that suits you.

Medication and pregnancy

Special conditions apply if you are pregnant, thinking of becoming pregnant, breast-feeding, or if you need to have an operation. When your medication is prescribed, always make sure you know as much as possible about how or when it should be taken and what side effects you might expect. Always tell any doctor or pharmacist advising or treating you that you are on medication for a heart condition. The British Heart Foundation, GUCH and Heart UK (contact details under Useful addresses, starting on page 95) all have lots of information about medication for heart conditions.

11

Heart surgery and rehabilitation

The idea of having heart surgery sounds alarming, but such great strides have been made in the treatment of heart conditions and in surgical techniques over the last twenty years that such surgery has almost become routine.

Surgery: an overview

In 2003, just under 30,000 people had coronary bypass surgery, where a surgeon grafts another blood vessel on to an artery, bypassing the damaged or narrowed section. Another 53,000 had what is known as 'percutaneous coronary intervention' or 'balloon angioplasty' in which a balloon containing a wire-mesh device called a 'stent' is inserted into the artery and then expanded. This squashes the fatty tissue which is blocking the artery and enables the blood to flow more freely. These are among the most common forms of cardiac surgery.

There are other operations you might have, for example to correct or replace faulty heart valves. We looked at valve problems in Chapter 2. If your heart valves don't open properly ('valve stenosis'), or don't close properly ('valve incompetence' or 'regurgitation'), blood will not flow as it should and your heart will be affected. Sometimes damaged heart valves can be repaired. In other cases they need to be replaced altogether, either by mechanical valves or animal valves from pigs or cows, also known as tissue valves.

If you have been diagnosed with some kinds of irregular heart rhythm, such as heart block or atrial fibrillation (see page 10), you may have to have a pacemaker fitted. This involves a short operation usually done under a local anaesthetic. A similar operation is used if you need to have an ICD or 'implantable cardioverter defibrillator' fitted. Like pacemakers, these devices are also used to correct specific abnormalities of the heart rhythm. They are usually fitted in those who have either had a heart attack or have cardiomyopathy. Both pacemakers and ICDs are also sometimes suitable for patients suffering from heart failure.

In cases of severe heart failure, either because of coronary heart disease or a condition such as cardiomyopathy, a patient might be recommended for a heart transplant. The first-ever heart transplant was carried out in South Africa in 1967. There were 128 transplants in the UK in 2002/3, plus 19 heart/lung transplants. Techniques are improving all the time and more effective immunosuppressant drugs mean there is less chance these days of a new heart being rejected. This means that people who in the past might not have been considered for a transplant can now be put on the waiting list. Sadly, there always far more patients waiting for heart and heart/lung transplants – indeed, for all organ transplants – than there are organs available. Better intensive care means that fewer people now die in road accidents. Six centres in the UK carry out heart transplants – Harefield near London, Papworth near Cambridge, the Queen Elizabeth Hospital in Birmingham, Wythenshawe Hospital in Manchester, the Freeman Hospital in Newcastle, and Glasgow Royal Infirmary.

Pacemakers

Pacemakers are fitted in people who have irregular heart rhythms or heart rates and also those who suffer from 'heart block' – a condition where the heart's normal electrical impulses are slowed down. The heart has its own natural pacemaker, a group of cells on the right side of the heart. If this doesn't work properly, an artificial pacemaker can be implanted instead.

There are several different kinds of pacemaker available. They consist of a tiny metal box, smaller than a matchbox, to which either one or two electrodes are attached, depending on the type of pacemaker. Which kind is prescribed for you will depend on your individual diagnosis.

The procedure

Most pacemakers are fitted by what is known as 'transvenous implantation', a procedure which takes between half an hour and one hour and is usually done under a local anaesthetic. The surgeon guides the lead into the correct part of the heart and the actual pacemaker fits into a 'pocket' between the skin and the chest muscle. An alternative procedure, called 'epicardial implantation', is when the lead is attached to the outer surface of the heart and the actual pacemaker is placed under the skin of the abdomen.

Having a pacemaker fitted usually involves staying in hospital for the night and taking it easy the following day. Most people can then return to their normal life. You will be given a pacemaker registration card and you should show this to any doctor or dentist who treats you in the future.

Living with a pacemaker

Having a pacemaker involves a very few lifestyle changes. For example you must inform the DLVA in Swansea if you are a driver. Drivers of LGVs or PCVs are not allowed to drive for three months after having pacemakers fitted. Car drivers should wait a week before driving again. When travelling by air, tell the operator of the security screening system that you have a heart pacemaker.

Most sports are permitted – it's important that you regain fitness after any heart surgery – though contact sports are not recommended as your pacemaker could be damaged.

Mobile phone users are advised to keep their phone at least six inches from their pacemaker and to use the opposite ear to the pacemaker when making and receiving calls. Don't keep your mobile in a pocket over the pacemaker! The British Heart Foundation has a booklet about pacemakers (contact details on page 95).

ICDs

ICDs, or 'implantable cardioverter defibrillators' are implanted in order to treat two different types of heart rhythm disturbance, called 'ventricular tachycardia' and 'ventricular fibrillation'. In the first of these, the cells in the lower chambers of the heart, the ventricles, produce electrical impulses which make the heart beat much too fast. Ventricular fibrillation is when the heart rhythm becomes so disorganized that the heart doesn't contract properly and isn't able to fulfil its normal pumping function. Both these conditions can be very serious and even fatal, so in suitable patients an ICD is implanted to correct the faulty heart rhythms.

An ICD consists of a small metal box, smaller than a matchbox, with one or two electrodes attached to it. It's used to monitor the heart rhythm. If it senses that there is a problem, it can deliver a series of small electrical impulses, known as pacing, to put things right. If this doesn't work it can give the heart a more serious shock to get it going again and restore normal rhythm.

The operation

The operation to insert an ICD is just a little more complex than inserting a pacemaker, but fairly similar. It can be done under either a local or a general anaesthetic and patients usually have to stay in the hospital cardiac unit for a couple of days. As with a pacemaker, the lead or leads are inserted into your heart and the pulse generator is implanted under the skin, usually just below the collarbone.

Your ICD should be tested before you leave hospital to make sure it's working properly. The team looking after you will tell you what sort of sensations to expect when the ICD delivers its treatment, ranging from mild palpitations to a 'thump' in the chest. They can also answer all your questions about living with an ICD, as can a booklet on the devices produced by the British Heart Foundation. There may be a local heart group you can join, enabling you to share your experiences with other patients with ICDs.

Living with an ICD

Again, some aspects of your life need to be adjusted if you have had an ICD implanted. You won't be allowed to drive a car for six months, and you won't be allowed to hold an LGV or PCV driving licence. While you will be advised to lead an active life, some activities are not recommended in case your ICD has to 'shock' you. Swimming on your own, ski-ing, climbing ladders and contact sports are best avoided. As with a pacemaker, it's best to keep your mobile phone away from your ICD; use the other ear and don't keep your phone in a breast pocket. Security devices at airports and other electro-magnetic fields can occasionally cause problems. Ask your cardiac team for advice on this or study the British Heart Foundation's ICD booklet. Always tell any medical professionals treating you that you have an ICD.

Coronary angioplasty

As we've seen, stable angina can often be controlled for many years with medication. Sometimes, though, your cardiologist may recommend what is known as 'revascularization treatment', which basically means surgery to widen the blocked arteries, or to bypass them altogether. An angiogram (see Chapter 10) will reveal where in your arteries the blockages are, and an angioplasty may then be advised in order to widen them and help the blood to flow through more freely.

Coronary angioplasty was first used in 1977 and has become a popular treatment for narrowed arteries, though it is not suitable for everyone with angina. It can be a planned operation, for those whose angina seems to be worsening. It can also be used after someone has had a heart attack or for a patient whose angina has become unstable.

The procedure

An angioplasty is usually carried out under a local anaesthetic. A catheter – a fine flexible tube – is passed, through an artery in your groin or arm, towards the coronary artery. When it reaches the narrowed part, the balloon on the end of the catheter is inflated to widen the artery. The catheter also contains a stainless-steel mesh 'stent' which then expands to hold the narrowed blood vessel open. The balloon is removed but the stent remains in place.

Stents

There are different types of stents. Some are coated with special drugs, and are used on particularly small arteries. More common are the uncoated types. Most of these operations work very well and blood flow improves, though sometimes the artery narrows again and angina symptoms return. In such cases, further treatment will be necessary, possibly in the form of bypass surgery. You will need to take anti-coagulant drugs like heparin and aspirin after the operation to prevent blood clots forming around the stent.

Aftercare

Many people have this operation as day cases, or you may be required to stay overnight. The cardiac team will tell you about aftercare, and may advise you to have someone take you home and stay with you for the first night. You shouldn't have any more chest pain. Tell the nurses and doctors if you do. Take it easy for a time. It's best to avoid carrying heavy shopping or children, for example, for at least a week. Don't drive for a week either. As with other heart operations, special rules apply if you have previously held an LGV or PCV driver's licence.

More information is available from your cardiac team, the hospital cardiac rehabilitation programme, the BHF and local patients' groups.

Coronary bypass surgery

Bypass surgery is just what it sounds like – a way of using healthy, unblocked blood vessels to bypass areas where the arteries are partly blocked by fatty deposits. The surgeon uses your own blood vessels for this procedure. Many patients have more than one bypass graft at once so that the effects of the operation last for as long as possible. Blood vessels are taken from other parts of the chest, the leg or the arm and grafted on to undamaged areas of the affected arteries.

Techniques

Usually, a heart-lung machine is used to circulate blood around the body while your surgeon operates on your heart. When the graft is complete and blood supply is restored, the heart begins to beat normally again. Traditionally a bypass operation is done through a cut down the middle of the breastbone, but some surgeons are now using smaller incisions, sometimes without the use of the heart-lung machine. Your own surgeon will be able to tell you about the techniques he is planning to use for your operation and why. New techniques like minimally invasive surgery are not available in every hospital or from every surgeon. Another new development is 'beating-heart' surgery – again, not yet available everywhere – which uses special equipment to stop part of the heart during the operation, rather than a conventional heart-lung machine.

Aftercare

As with all major operations, you can expect some post-operative pain in your chest and also in your leg or arm where the replacement blood vessel was removed. You will probably be able to sit out of bed a day or two after your operation and go home in about a week. It may be as long as two or three months before you can return to work, depending on your job.

Coronary bypass surgery is very effective in stopping the pain of angina caused by furred-up arteries. However there is always the possibility of the new 'arteries' furring up again if you don't change the lifestyle that led to the problem in the first place. If you haven't already given up smoking and taken steps with diet or medication to control your cholesterol levels and blood pressure, it's even more important that you do so now. If your angina does return, you may have to have further heart surgery.

The BHF booklet, *Coronary Angioplasty and Coronary Bypass Surgery*, is worth reading if you are recommended to have one or other of these procedures. In some cases, either one might be suitable for you. Your cardiac team will help you to make an informed choice.

Future developments

There are new developments in heart surgery all the time. New approaches like gene therapy might, in future, enable new, healthy blood vessels to grow, or new heart muscle cells might be able to replace those damaged by a heart attack or a condition like cardiomyopathy. Trials of blood vessels grown from patients' own skin cells are taking place in both the USA and at Papworth Hospital in Cambridge.

Heart valve surgery

Some people are born with faulty heart valves; others develop faults after illnesses like rheumatic fever, or simply later in life. Faulty heart valves sometimes cause no problems at all, or they can cause breathlessness, dizziness, fainting, shortness of breath and swelling of the legs and ankles as well as chest pain. An ECG, chest X-ray and/or echocardiogram may reveal heart valve problems. Drugs such as ACE inhibitors, diuretics and digoxin are sometimes prescribed, but if symptoms are not relieved or recur, surgery may be recommended.

Balloon treatment

'Balloon treatment' or, more technically 'mitral valvuloplasty' is a way of stretching the mitral valve if it's not opening properly. The technique is similar to angioplasty as it involves the insertion of a catheter with a balloon on the end which stretches the valve. This is a relatively minor procedure, but is not often suitable for other valves. Leaking mitral valves can also sometimes be repaired.

Mechanical valves

Valve replacement involves removing the damaged or malfunctioning valve altogether and replacing it with a new one. Most often, mechanical valves are used. There are different types, which are made of carbon fibre, and make a clicking sound when they open and close. This can be disconcerting if you're not used to it! If you have a mechanical heart valve fitted you will also be prescribed anti-coagulant drugs to prevent the formation of clots around the new valve.

Tissue valves

Another type of valve is a 'tissue valve' made from animal tissue – pigs or cows – or occasionally even human tissue. It sounds a bit like science fiction but they are as effective as mechanical valves and don't make the clicking noise. Patients with tissue valves may only have to take anti-coagulants for a short time. However they tend to wear out more quickly than mechanical valves. You will probably want to discuss the type of valve you have with your cardiac surgeon.

Avoiding infection

There is a slight possibility of infection in patients who have had replacement valves. You will be advised to take antibiotics if you have dental treatment or surgery and asked to take special care of your teeth and gums. This is because infections can easily enter the bloodstream via the gums and cause a serious inflammation of the heart called endocarditis. The BHF also recommend that if you have an inter-uterine contraceptive device (or coil) fitted after you have had a valve replaced, you should also take a course of antibiotics.

Heart transplants

Heart transplants are usually carried out on patients with severe heart failure. Less often, those with abnormal heart valves or congenital heart abnormalities will be recommended for a transplant. As there is always a waiting list for transplant surgery because of the shortage of donors, other ways of treating heart failure will be tried before a transplant is suggested.

Not everyone with heart failure is suitable for a transplant. You need to be assessed at one of the UK's six transplant centres to find out whether you are suitable. There are risks, and the job of the transplant team is to find out whether you will benefit. Some of the issues to be considered are:

- whether you have any infection which, however minor, could become life-threatening when you are taking the vital immuno-suppressant drugs;
- how well your liver and kidneys are functioning, as the immunosuppressant drug cyclosporin can cause kidney damage;
- whether the pressure in your pulmonary artery (which leads to your lungs) is too high. If it is, a donor heart might not be able to cope and may fail. If this is the case you may be eligible for a heart-lung transplant instead.

Depending on the results of your assessment you may be placed on the waiting list for a transplant. This is a tense time as of course you have no idea when, or if, a heart will become available. If your heart failure is extremely severe you may be in hospital. You will certainly need to be contactable at all times. The transplant team and your cardiologist will explain the procedure if a donor heart is found, and there are also support groups like the Transplant Support Network (contact details on page 99).

If a donor heart becomes available you will need further tests and checks and the team will also need to know that the donor heart is suitable for you.

The operation

A heart transplant operation lasts between three and five hours. As with other heart operations, you will be taken from the operating theatre to intensive care until your condition has stabilized. Once all is well you may be moved to a high-dependency ward or a special area in a cardiac ward. Because of the risk of infection you will be cared for after your operation in a separate room or bay, and will only be allowed to receive a small number of visitors at first.

Afterwards

After the transplant you will find you have to take large numbers of drugs. There are the immunosuppressants such as cyclosporin, azathioprine and prednisolone, which prevent your body rejecting the new organ. You will also be on antibiotics to prevent infection, drugs to lower your blood pressure and possibly diuretics to prevent water retention. It's important that you take all your drugs as directed.

Transplant patients usually have to stay in hospital for two or three weeks, and in accommodation close to the transplant centre for a month or two. After this there will be weekly outpatient appointments for a time. You will need to be carefully monitored at regular intervals by the transplant centre for months or even years. As with all heart surgery, rehabilitation is very important. You'll be given advice on a healthy diet and lifestyle, including exercise. Normally you're recommended not to do any heavy work for six weeks after the operation, but as time passes you will find you can return to a normal life. Many transplant patients take part in sports and games and most are recommended a minimum of 30 minutes' moderate exercise every day. You're advised not to go swimming for a year after your transplant. This is because of the possibility of infection.

There are other lifestyle issues too. You're not required to tell the DVLA about your transplant, but you shouldn't drive for three months after the operation and you will need to inform your car insurance company. Vaccinations are not always safe because of the drugs you are taking, and you should be as careful as you can to avoid any kind of infection. Pay special attention to dental hygiene and tell your dentist you have had a transplant. It's advisable to avoid high-risk foods like unpasteurized cheeses and raw eggs in case of food poisoning. The transplant team and patients' groups can give advice on all lifestyle issues after your transplant and you should also read the BHF booklet on the subject.

Rehabilitation

You'll probably feel weak and possibly quite nervous while you are recovering from heart surgery of any kind. It's important that you don't try to do too much and that you get plenty of rest, but on the other hand you do need to get back to a normal, healthy lifestyle. You should be told in hospital about how much you should be doing when you return home. If no one tells you, ask!

If you've had a heart attack, for example, the cardiac team should refer you to a rehabilitation programme, either at the hospital or at another nearby centre. You may be invited to go once or twice a week for six to eight weeks or even longer. Don't be tempted to miss out on this as it's an important part of your treatment. As well as advising you on medical issues, the programme can also increase your confidence, relieve any anxieties you may have about taking up normal living again, and introduce you to others who have been through the same kind of experiences as you have. If you are not referred for rehab, contact the BHF for advice.

Most cardiac rehabiliation programmes include help with:

- exercise. You'll be personally assessed and a programme of exercise will be worked out for you, including a warm-up routine, aerobic exercises to keep your heart and lungs as fit as possible, and cool-down exercises. You may well end up fitter than before!
- relaxation. Stress is an enemy of heart health and heart disease and/or hospital treatment is stressful in itself. There are lots of ways you can learn to relax (see Chapter 9) and your rehab programme may incorporate some of these.
- topics like healthy eating, risk factors for heart disease, giving up smoking, practical issues like driving and going back to work, and personal relationships. It's not always easy for the partners and families of women with heart disease. They too suffer from stress and anxiety and may be anxious to help without really knowing what they can do. The rehab team will be able to advise you.

Some women are reluctant to ask about resuming a sex life but it's a common question for heart patients and the BHF have a video on the subject. Once you're well enough to resume normal life and exercise, gentle love-making can only do you good! Joining a rehabilitation programme and heart patients' support groups can help to convince you that there *is* life after heart disease.

Useful addresses and further reading

Bach Flower Remedies
The Dr Edward Bach Centre
Mount Vernon
Bakers Lane
Brightwell-cum-Sotwell
Oxon OX10 0PZ
Tel.: 01491 834678
Website: www.bachcentre.com

Blood Pressure Association
60 Cranmer Terrace
London SW17 0QS
Tel.: 020 8772 4994
Website: www.bpassoc.org.uk

British Autogenic Society
C/o The Royal London Homeoepathic Hospital
60 Great Ormond Street
London WC1N 3HR
Tel.: 020 7391 8888
Website: www.autogenic-therapy.org.uk
Email: admin@autogenic-therapy.org.uk

British Complementary Medicine Association
PO Box 5122
Bournemouth BH8 0WG
Tel.: 0845 345 5977
Website: www.bcma.co.uk

British Heart Foundation
14 Fitzhardinge Street
London W1H 6DH
Heart Information Line: 0845 0 70 80 70 (9 am to 5 pm, Monday to
    Friday)
Website: www.bhf.org.uk

Email: internet@bhf.org.uk
BHF statistics website: www.heartstats.org

British Homeopathic Association
Hahnemann House
29 Park Street West
Luton LU1 3BE
Tel.: 0870 444 3950
Website: www.trusthomeopathy.org

British Society of Clinical Hypnosis
Tel.: 01262 403103
Website: www.bsch.org.uk
Email: sec@bsch.org.uk

British Wheel of Yoga
25 Jermyn Street
Sleaford
Lincs NG34 7RU
Tel.: 01529 306851
Website: www.bwy.org.uk
Email: office@bwy.org.uk

Cardiomyopathy Association
40 The Metro Centre
Tolpits Lane
Watford WD18 9SB
Tel.: 01923 249977
Helpline: 0800 018 1024
Website: www.cardiomyopathy.org
Email: info@cardiomyopathy.org

Diabetes UK
Macleod House
10 Parkway
London NW1 7AA
Information Line: 0845 120 2960
Website: www.diabetes.org.uk
Email: info@diabetes.org.uk

Fitness First
Support Centre
58 Fleets Lane
Poole
Dorset BH15 3BT
Tel.: 0870 898 80 80 (general enquiries)
Website: www.fitnessfirst.co.uk

GUCH (Grown Up Congenital Heart Patients Association)
75 Tuddenham Avenue
Ipswich
Suffolk IP4 2HG
Helpline: 0800 854 759
Website: www.guch.org.uk

Heart Research UK
Suite 12D
Joseph's Well
Leeds LS3 1AB
Tel.: 0113 234 7474
Website: www.heartresearch.org.uk
Email: info@heartresearch.org.uk

Heart UK (the cholesterol charity)
7 North Road
Maidenhead
Berks SL6 1PE
Tel.: 01628 628 638
Website: www.heartuk.org.uk
Email: md@heartuk.org.uk

International Stress Management Association
PO Box 26
South Petherton
Somerset TA13 5WY
Tel.: 07000 780430
Website: www.isma.org.uk

Marfan Association UK
Rochester House

5 Aldershot Road
Fleet
Hants GU51 3NG
Tel.: 01252 810472
Website: www.marfan.org.uk

The Menopause Exchange
PO Box 205
Bushey
Herts WD23 1ZS
Tel.: 020 8420 7245
Email: norma@menopause-exchange.co.uk

National Institute of Medical Herbalists
Elm House
54 Mary Arches Street
Exeter EX4 3BA
Tel.: 01392 426022
Website: www.nimh.org.uk
Email: nimh@ukexeter.freeserve.co.uk

Natural Health Advisory Service/Women's Nutrition Clinic
PO Box 268
Lewes
East Sussex BN7 1QN
Tel.: 01273 487366
Website: www.naturalhealthas.com

Specializes in women's general health matters.

NHS Stop Smoking
Helpline: 0800 169 0 169
Website: www.givingupsmoking.co.uk

No Panic
93 Brands Farm Way
Telford
TF3 2JQ
Helpline: 0808 808 0545 (10 am to 10 pm, 365 days a year)
Helpline from outside UK: 0044 1952 590545
Website: www.nopanic.org.uk

QUIT (help for stopping smoking)
Helpline: 0800 00 22 00
Website: www.quit.org.uk

Slimming World
PO Box 55
Alfreton
Derbyshire DE55 4UE
Tel.: 0870 330 7733
Website: www.slimming-world.com

Sport England
Tel.: 08458 508 508
Website: www.sportengland.org

Sport Scotland
Tel.: 0131 317 7200
Website: www.sportscotland.org.uk

Sports Council for Wales
Tel.: 0845 045 0904
Website: www.sports-council-wales.co.uk

T'ai Chi Finder Ltd
21 The Avenue
London E11 2EE
Tel.: 0845 8900 744
Website: www.taichifinder.co.uk
Please contact via post, telephone or website form: no personal callers.

Transcendental Meditation
Information Line: 08705 143733
Website: www.t-m.org.uk

Transplant Support Network
223 Temple Row
Keighley
West Yorkshire BD21 2AH
Support Lines: 0800 027 4490/4491

Website: www.transplantsupportnetwork.org.uk
Email: tsn@btconnect.com

UK Transplant Service
Fox Den Road
Stoke Gifford
Bristol BS4 8RR
Donor Line: 0845 60 60 400
Website: www.uktransplant.org.uk

Vegetarian Society of the United Kingdom
Parkdale
Dunham Road
Altrincham
Cheshire WA14 4QG
Tel.: 0161 925 2000 (8.30 am to 5 pm, Monday to Friday)
Website: www.vegsoc.org

Weight Watchers
Tel.: 08457 123 000
Website: www.weightwatchers.co.uk

Other useful websites

www.food.gov.uk – information on healthy eating
www.activeplaces.com – type in your postcode for local information
  about sporting facilities
www.everydaysport.com

Further reading

Alexander, Jane, *The Overload Solution*. Piatkus, London, 2005 – on
  stress management.
Atkinson, Mary, *A Practical Guide to Self-Massage for Health and
  Vitality*. Cico Books, London, 2005.
Stewart, Maryon, *Beat Menopause Naturally*. Natural Health Pub-
  lishing, c/o Natural Health Advisory Service, Lewes, 2003.

Index

ACE inhibitors 62, 79–80, 82–3, 90
acupuncture 31
aerobic exercise 43
alcohol 21, 40–1, 67
alpha blockers 79
angina 6–8, 17, 48–50, 81–2, 87
angioplasty 2, 17, 87–9
angiotensin II blockers 62, 79, 82
anti-arrhythmia drugs 82–3
anti-coagulant drugs 83
anti-platelet drugs 82
anxiety 66
arrhythmia 9–10, 82
ASCOT study 79
aspirin 82
atherosclerosis 4
atrial fibrillation 10, 84
atrium 3, 9–10
autogenic training 73

Bach flower remedies 72
balloon angioplasty 84
balloon treatment 90
beta-blockers 79–80, 81–2
binge-drinking 21, 41
Blood Pressure Association 79, 95
body mass index (BMI) 34
British Heart Foundation (BHF) ix, 16, 17,
    21, 26, 49, 51, 57, 60, 65, 67, 83, 90,
    91, 93–4

calcium-channel blockers 79–80, 81–2
cardiac enzyme tests 77
cardiomyopathy 4, 9, 10–13, 48, 84–5
Cardiomyopathy Association 13
centrally acting hypertensives 79
cholesterol 5, 13, 17, 20–2, 25, 35–6, 37–9,
    44, 55–6, 58, 61, 66, 80–1, 90
clot-busting drugs 82
congenital heart disease 53–4
contraception 51–2
coronary angiogram 78, 88
coronary artery 3
coronary artery bypass 2, 17, 84, 89–90
coronary care unit (CCU) 9
coronary heart disease (CHD) ix, 1, 10, 13,
    20, 23, 44, 51, 59, 67, 75, 85

death rates ix–x
dental hygiene 14, 93
depression 66
diabetes 21, 44, 51, 59–64
Diabetes UK 21, 61–2, 96
diet 1, 19, 75, 90
digoxin 82–3, 90
diuretics 79–80, 82–3, 90, 93

echocardiogram 12, 15, 76, 90
electrocardiogram (ECG) 6, 12, 75, 90
electrocardiograph 2
electrophysiological testing 77
endocarditis 14–15
endothelium 4
exercise x, 1, 20, 42–50, 62, 75
    for heart patients 48–50, 93–4

familial combined hyperlipidaemia 13
familial hypercholesterolaemia 13
family history 17
fats 35–6
fibrates 80–1
fight-or-flight syndrome 66
Framingham Study 1

glyceryl trinitrate (GTN) spray 7, 48, 50,
    81
Grown-Up Congenital Heart Patients
    Association (GUCH) 15, 54, 83, 97

healthy drinking guidelines 41
healthy eating 33–41, 94
heart attack ix, 1, 4, 5, 6, 9, 17, 20, 48, 51,
    56, 60, 66, 82, 84
    symptoms of 4, 5, 17
heart block 10, 84–5
heart failure 8, 49, 82, 84–5, 91
    symptoms of 8
heart-lung transplant 85, 92
heart surgery 2
heart transplant 2, 85, 91–3
Heart UK 39, 83, 97
herbal medicine 72
high blood pressure 5, 17, 21, 41, 42, 44,
    49, 51, 61, 67–8, 75, 78, 90

homocysteine 40
homoeopathy 72
hormone replacement therapy (HRT) 54–7, 63
hormones 20–1, 51–8
hypnotherapy 31, 73
hypoglycaemia 62

immunosuppressant drugs 92
implantable cardioverter defibrillator (ICD) 11, 12, 84, 86–7
incompetence (of heart valves) 14, 84
insomnia 68

life expectancy 1
low blood pressure 68

Marfan Association 14, 97
Marfan syndrome 13–14
massage 73
maximum heart rate (MHR) 43
mechanical valves 91
meditation 73
menopause 6, 20, 51–2, 54–8
mono-unsaturated fats 36
MRI scan 77
myocardial infarction (MI) 4

Natural Health Advisory Service/Women's Nutrition Clinic 98
nicotine replacement therapy (NRT) 31
nitrates 81

obesity x, 19, 33, 41, 42, 51, 59, 61, 67
oestrogen 51, 55–6
open-heart surgery 2

pacemaker 9–10, 84–6
panic attacks 74
passive smoking 26
percutaneous coronary intervention 84
periodontal disease 22
PET scan 77
Pill, the 51–2
poly-unsaturated fats 36
potassium channel activators 81–2
pregnancy 52–4

radionuclide tests 77

rehabilitation 48, 93–4
relaxation 94
resins 80–1
resting heart rate (RHR) 43
risk factors 19–22

saturated fats 35
sex 49, 94
smoking x, 1, 19, 21, 23–32, 42, 51, 61, 67, 75, 90
   giving up 26–32, 94
   and weight gain 28–9
social support, lack of 66
soya 58
statins 80–1
stem cell research 2
stenosis 14, 48, 84
stent 2, 84, 88
stress 21, 65–74, 94
stress-busters 70–4
symptoms of heart attack 4
   in women 5, 17
symptoms of heart failure 8

t'ai chi 73
tissue valves 91
trans fats 36
triglycerides 39–40, 55, 80–1
'Type A personality' 66

valve surgery 90–1
valves 3, 4, 14
valvular heart disease 14, 83
vegetarians 37
veins 3
ventricles 3
ventricular fibrillation 86
ventricular tachycardia 86

waist-to-hip ratio (WHR) 28, 34
Women's Nutrition Clinic 57–8, 63
   see also Natural Advisory Service
work stress 65

X-rays 76, 90

yoga 72

Zyban 31